Multiple Choice Questions
in Regional Anaesthesia

369 0246408

Rajesh Gupta   Dilip Patel

Multiple Choice Questions in Regional Anaesthesia

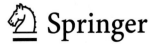 Springer

WO 300 GUP

Rajesh Gupta, MD, FRCA, EDRA
Department of Anaesthesia
Royal Free Hospital
London
UK

Dilip Patel, FRCA
Department of Anaesthesia
Royal Free Hospital
London
UK

McINDOE HANDS HOSPITAL
LIBRARY
MONKSCOURT AVENUE
AIRDRIE ML60 US
01236 712005

3690246402
£ 25.64
10|4|13

ISBN 978-3-642-31256-4   ISBN 978-3-642-31257-1   (eBook)
DOI 10.1007/978-3-642-31257-1
Springer Heidelberg New York Dordrecht London

Library of Congress Control Number: 2012947658

© Springer-Verlag Berlin Heidelberg 2013
This work is subject to copyright. All rights are reserved by the Publisher, whether the whole or part of the material is concerned, specifically the rights of translation, reprinting, reuse of illustrations, recitation, broadcasting, reproduction on microfilms or in any other physical way, and transmission or information storage and retrieval, electronic adaptation, computer software, or by similar or dissimilar methodology now known or hereafter developed. Exempted from this legal reservation are brief excerpts in connection with reviews or scholarly analysis or material supplied specifically for the purpose of being entered and executed on a computer system, for exclusive use by the purchaser of the work. Duplication of this publication or parts thereof is permitted only under the provisions of the Copyright Law of the Publisher's location, in its current version, and permission for use must always be obtained from Springer. Permissions for use may be obtained through RightsLink at the Copyright Clearance Center. Violations are liable to prosecution under the respective Copyright Law.
The use of general descriptive names, registered names, trademarks, service marks, etc. in this publication does not imply, even in the absence of a specific statement, that such names are exempt from the relevant protective laws and regulations and therefore free for general use.
While the advice and information in this book are believed to be true and accurate at the date of publication, neither the authors nor the editors nor the publisher can accept any legal responsibility for any errors or omissions that may be made. The publisher makes no warranty, express or implied, with respect to the material contained herein.

Printed on acid-free paper

Springer is part of Springer Science+Business Media (www.springer.com)

Contents

1 Benefits and Complications

1. The benefits of regional anaesthesia:
   (a) Better quality of analgesia
   (b) Prolonged duration of analgesia
   (c) Other perioperative benefits than analgesia
   (d) Minimal effect on autonomic system
   (e) Decreased hospital stay

2. Regional anaesthesia is known to decrease:
   (a) Blood loss
   (b) Complications after vascular surgery
   (c) Shivering after induction of anaesthesia
   (d) Complications after colon surgery
   (e) Morbidity and mortality associated with general anaesthesia

3. Changes in cardiovascular system seen with pain are:
   (a) Increased catecholamine increase
   (b) Decreased myocardial oxygen demand
   (c) Bradycardia
   (d) Hypertension
   (e) Decreased risk of thrombotic complications

4. All are seen in pulmonary system with pain:
   (a) Increased vital capacity
   (b) Increased functional residual capacity
   (c) Decreased tidal volume
   (d) Increased chest infections
   (e) Impaired cough

R. Gupta, D. Patel, *Multiple Choice Questions in Regional Anaesthesia*,
DOI 10.1007/978-3-642-31257-1_1, © Springer-Verlag Berlin Heidelberg 2013

5. Following are seen in stress response to surgery:
   (a) Increased catabolism
   (b) Decreased anabolism
   (c) Decreased sodium and water retention
   (d) Weight loss
   (e) No effect on muscle protein

6. Regional anaesthesia:
   (a) Improves pulmonary function
   (b) Prevents sympathetic activation
   (c) Decreases paralytic ileus following abdominal
       procedures
   (d) Decreases incidence of thrombotic complications
       in upper abdominal procedures
   (e) Improves cardiac performance and may even have
       beneficial effects on the oxygen delivery/demand
       ratio

7. Endocrine changes in stress response:
   (a) Concentration of all anterior pituitary hormones
       is increased during surgery.
   (b) Both ACTH and cortisol secretion is increased.
   (c) Growth hormone secretion is related to severity of
       injury.
   (d) Insulin is anabolic.
   (e) Testosterone concentrations are decreased for several
       days after surgery.

8. Regional anaesthesia affects endocrine system:
   (a) Prolactin secretion is decreased.
   (b) Sympathetic response to surgery is not blocked.
   (c) Thyroid hormone secretion is not affected.
   (d) Hyperglycaemic response to surgery is not
       blocked.
   (e) Oxygen consumption is increased after surgery.

9. Modifications of stress response seen with regional anaesthesia:
   (a) Neurogenic stimuli are blocked from surgical area to central nervous system and endocrine system.
   (b) Involves both afferent and efferent neurogenic pathways.
   (c) Hyperglycaemic response is mediated by both afferent and efferent pathways.
   (d) There is a known mechanism for cortical response.
   (e) Efferent sympathetic pathway blockade to liver may be important in pancreatic islet response.

10. Preoperative preparation for regional anaesthesia:
    (a) Written consent is not necessary.
    (b) All complications however minor should be informed during the consent.
    (c) Intravenous sedation can be used for sedation.
    (d) Full investigations are not required as for general anaesthesia.

11. Complications associated with regional anaesthesia can be decreased by:
    (a) Appropriate informed consent
    (b) Physician-patient communication
    (c) Post-operative follow-up visit
    (d) Accurate and meticulous documentation
    (e) Preoperative patient selection

12. All are absolute contraindications for regional anaesthesia:
    (a) Patient refusal
    (b) Lack of nerve stimulator
    (c) Lack of resuscitation facilities
    (d) Coagulopathy
    (e) INR > 2 in ophthalmic procedures

13. Monitoring in regional anaesthesia:
     (a) Needle phobia is seen in 15 % of patients.
     (b) Only ECG is required as a standard.
     (c) Baseline blood pressure should be recorded before starting regional anaesthesia.
     (d) Assistant should observe and aid patient all the time.
     (e) Clinical guidelines for discharge should be met before discharge.

14. Anticoagulants in regional anaesthesia:
     (a) A single dose of warfarin causes prolongation of prothrombin time in 100 % patients.
     (b) Patients with acute thromboembolic disease exhibit heparin resistance.
     (c) Enhanced prothrombin time response is seen in males.
     (d) Fondaparinux has a half-life of 20 h.
     (e) Subcutaneous heparin is safest among anticoagulants in incidence of spinal hematomas.

15. Effects seen with thoracic epidural:
     (a) Loss of ionotropic and chronotropic drive to myocardium.
     (b) Stroke volume and cardiac output are not altered.
     (c) Chest pain is relieved in coronary artery disease and angina pectoris.
     (d) Pulmonary function is improved after cardiac surgery.
     (e) Attenuates mean arterial pressure during laryngoscopy.

16. Spinal hematoma after regional anaesthesia:
     (a) Seen more after epidural anaesthesia than spinal anaesthesia.
     (b) Are symptomatic immediately after surgery.

(c) Cauda equine is relatively immune to compression effects of hematoma.
(d) Is seen more in females.
(e) Spontaneous hematomas seen more with LMWH than thrombolytic therapy.

17. Nerve injuries due to needle trauma in peripheral nerve block:
    (a) Incidence is 1–2 %.
    (b) Most common is axonotmesis.
    (c) Most cases settle by 3 months.
    (d) Mostly is seen due to needle trauma and injection pressure.
    (e) Not seen if performed in awake patients.

18. Nerve injuries due to needle trauma:
    (a) Small-gauge needles are less likely to damage nerves than larger gauge.
    (b) Blunt needles are better than sharp-end needles.
    (c) Sterilising agents and preservatives can cause neurotoxicity.
    (d) Addition of vasoconstrictor to local anaesthetic may enhance the damage caused by an intraneural injection.
    (e) Can be avoided by limiting pressure of injection.

19. Nerve injuries:
    (a) Nerve conduction studies test the function of large sensory and motor nerve fibres.
    (b) EMG is used to evaluate small motor units.
    (c) Brown-Sequard syndrome is a complication of interscalene block.
    (d) Patient positioning is a significant factor in nerve injuries.
    (e) Signs of symptoms of spinal cord compression must be dealt with urgently.

20. Pneumothorax seen with regional anaesthesia:
    (a) Seen more with supraclavicular technique than interscalene.
    (b) The incidence is equal on both the sides.
    (c) Ultrasonography prevents it totally.
    (d) Patient may not become symptomatic until 20 % pneumothorax is present.
    (e) Risk is reduced in vertical techniques.

21. Horner's syndrome includes:
    (a) Ipsilateral miosis
    (b) Ptosis
    (c) Exophthalmos
    (d) Loss of sweating
    (e) Enophthalmos.

22. Phrenic nerve palsy during supraclavicular nerve block:
    (a) Seen in 100 % of patients with interscalene brachial plexus block.
    (b) Is purely a motor nerve.
    (c) Permanent nerve palsy is never seen.
    (d) Decrease in FVC, FEV1 and PEF is seen on lung function tests.
    (e) Advanced pulmonary disease is a contradiction to bilateral supraclavicular techniques.

23. Preoperative assessment for regional anaesthesia:
    (a) Risk of local anaesthetic toxicity is increased in patients with right to left shunts.
    (b) Local anaesthetics should be used cautiously in sick sinus syndrome.
    (c) High spinal anaesthesia can cause anti-peristaltic movements and gastric regurgitation.
    (d) Lignocaine should be avoided in patients with glucose-6-phosphate dehydrogenase deficiency.
    (e) Lidocaine is contraindicated in malignant hyperthermia.

24. Brainstem anaesthesia seen with ophthalmic blocks:
    (a) Symptoms can occur immediately on injection.
    (b) Short globe axial length is a risk factor.
    (c) Diagnosis is by fundoscopic examination.
    (d) Aiming the needle between inferior and lateral rectus can help avoid the complication.
    (e) Incidence is 1:350–1,500 ophthalmic cases.

25. Anticoagulants:
    (a) No increase risk in hematoma is seen if interval of 4 h is given between dose and catheter insertion or removal.
    (b) Dose should be given 6 h after the catheter insertion or removal.
    (c) Infusion if given for more than 14 days should be monitored for heparin-induced thrombocytopenia.
    (d) An interval of 10–12 h would be given after needle placement or catheter removal if low molecular weight heparin is used.
    (e) Enoxaparin can be used for up to 40 mg/day safely.

26. Effects of epidural anaesthesia on cardiorespiratory system:
    (a) FEV1 and FVC are decreased.
    (b) Increase in functional residual capacity.
    (c) Decreased risk of thrombotic complications.
    (d) Increased PO_2.
    (e) Better pain control in cardiac surgery.

27. Pulmonary effects seen with regional anaesthesia:
    (a) Post-operative complications are decreased.
    (b) Lung volumes are altered.
    (c) Both FEV1 and FVC are decreased in interscalene block.
    (d) Paravertebral block improves arterial oxygen saturation and peak expiratory flow rate better than epidural.

28. Effect of regional anaesthesia on renal system:
    (a) Blood flow to kidneys is increased in low thoracic neuraxial anaesthesia.
    (b) Acidemia in chronic renal failure can cause bupivacaine toxicity.
    (c) Hyperkalemia decreases toxicity of bupivacaine.
    (d) Increased risk of toxicity in peripheral nervous system in chronic renal failure.
    (e) Haemodialysis removes lidocaine effectively.

29. Effects seen with regional anaesthesia in renal dysfunction:
    (a) Alpha-1-acid glycoprotein levels increase in uraemia.
    (b) Onset time and duration of anaesthesia is decreased in patients with uraemia.
    (c) Uraemic patients are at higher risk for thrombotic events.
    (d) Both general anaesthesia and regional anaesthesia are equally effective in improving blood flow through AV fistula.
    (e) Dysfunction in platelet structure is seen in uraemia.

30. Regional anaesthesia in hepatic dysfunction:
    (a) Local anaesthetic toxicity is increased.
    (b) Dosages should be increased to cause the same effect.
    (c) Grape juice can increase amide local anaesthetic toxicity.
    (d) Regional anaesthesia has no effect on portal blood flow.
    (e) Drugs inhibiting microsomal enzymes increase toxicity.

31. Regional anaesthesia and endocrine system:
    (a) More risk of ischaemia of nerves in diabetes mellitus.

(b) Nerve stimulator is reliable for electro location of nerves in diabetes mellitus.
(c) Regional anaesthesia ameliorates hypoglycaemic response to surgery.
(d) Double crush syndrome is seen in nerve entrapment.
(e) Higher block heights may be seen in obese patients.

32. Coagulation factors:
    (a) Factor VII has the longest half-life.
    (b) Normal INR means all factors are present in adequate levels.
    (c) A factor level of 40 % is sufficient for haemostasis.
    (d) INR < 1.2 is required for effective haemostasis.
    (e) Usage of garlic decreases factor VII (F).

33. Antiplatelet medications:
    (a) Ticlodipine causes irreversible inhibition of platelets.
    (b) Clopidogrel should be stopped for 14 days prior to regional anaesthesia.
    (c) Abciximab has a duration of 48 h.
    (d) Eptifibatide and tiorfan belong to same category of anticoagulant drugs.
    (e) Ginko is known to inhibit platelet-activating factor.

34. Epidural abscess after dural puncture:
    (a) *Streptococci* is the most common organism.
    (b) Most common cause is epidural catheter.
    (c) Steroid administration protects against the abscess formation.
    (d) Immunocompromised patients are at increased risk.
    (e) Conservative management shows best results.

35.   Infections in immunocompromised patients:
   (a)   Lidocaine and bupivacaine show dose-related
         inhibition of microorganisms.
   (b)   Opioids inhibit microorganisms more than local
         anaesthetics.
   (c)   Catheter hub accounts for the majority of infections
         in immunocompromised.
   (d)   Bacterial filter effectively prevents infections.
   (e)   Multiple catheter placements is a risk factor.

36.   Infectious complications in peripheral nerve blocks:
   (a)   *S. epidermidis* is the most common organism
         colonising the catheters.
   (b)   Male gender is a risk factor.
   (c)   Presence of fever was seen a strong predictor
         of colonisation.

37.   Hypotension in regional anaesthesia:
   (a)   Local anaesthetics cause a dose-dependent negative
         ionotropic effect on cardiac muscle.
   (b)   Clonidine causes hypotension by blocking alpha 2
         receptors.
   (c)   Bezold-Jarisch reflex can contribute to it.
   (d)   Interscalene block can cause hypotension in
         shoulder surgery.
   (e)   Elevated body mass index is a risk factor.

38.   Cardiac arrest during regional anaesthesia:
   (a)   Seen more with spinal anaesthesia than epidural
         or peripheral nerve block.
   (b)   Hip replacement surgery is a known risk factor
         for cardiac arrest.
   (c)   Volume loading prior to spinal can prevent
         hypotension and cardiac arrest.
   (d)   Colloids are better than crystalloids in preventing
         hypotension-induced cardiac arrest.
   (e)   Arrests involved with regional anaesthesia are
         primarily hypoxic in origin.

39. Toxicity seen with local anaesthetics:
    (a) More seen with R (+) isomer than S (−) isomer.
    (b) Inadequate production of cAMP accounts for refractoriness of bupivacaine CV toxicity to standard resuscitation measures.
    (c) Lidocaine produces arrhythmias more than bupivacaine.
    (d) True allergy to local anaesthetics is most commonly seen with ropivacaine.
    (e) CNS toxicity manifests earlier than CV toxicity.

40. Central nervous system toxicity seen with local anaesthetics:
    (a) Is an outcome of loss of inhibition of excitatory pathways in the CNS.
    (b) Metallic taste is a frequent accompaniment.
    (c) Acidosis is protective against convulsive effects.
    (d) CC/CNS ratio is least for ropivacaine.
    (e) Origin of seizures is from amygdale.

41. Epinephrine used as an adjuvant:
    (a) Extends block duration, limits systemic uptake, supplements analgesic effect, and acts as an indicator of intravascular injection.
    (b) Can cause toxicity to peripheral nerves in patients with diabetes or chemotherapy.
    (c) Local anaesthetics and epinephrine have no effect on peripheral nerve blood flow.
    (d) Epidural usage can increase cardiac output.
    (e) Can aggravate local anaesthetic-induced neuraxial or peripheral nerve injury.

42. Adjuvants in regional anaesthesia:
    (a) Clonidine inhibits firing of wide dynamic range neurons in spinal dorsal column.
    (b) Neostigmine works supraspinally if given intrathecal.

(c) Ketamine is a NMDA receptor antagonist.
(d) Magnesium prolongs fentanyl intrathecal analgesia.
(e) Midazolam has minimal neurotoxicity if given intrathecal.

43. Transient neurologic symptoms after neuraxial block:
   (a) Symptoms begin as soon as local anaesthetic is injected.
   (b) Pain is mostly seen in the back.
   (c) Symptoms can take up to 4 days to resolve.
   (d) Diagnosis is by neurologic findings on examination.
   (e) Daily functional activities are not hampered.

44. Peripheral nerve injury:
   (a) Wallerian degeneration occurs proximally to injury.
   (b) Retrograde degeneration occurs proximally to the site of injury.
   (c) Swelling of cytoplasm indicates severe injury.
   (d) Nissl substance is an indicator of recovery.
   (e) Axonal regeneration takes about 1 week to start.

45. Risk factors for peripheral nerve injury:
   (a) For "double crush injury", the second insult should be along the peripheral nerve trunk.
   (b) There are no known surgical risk factors.
   (c) Most common surgical risk factor is direct surgical trauma.
   (d) Most injuries causing motor deficit have a surgical cause.
   (e) Local anaesthetics can cause neural damage.

46. Management of post-operative nerve dysfunction:
   (a) Baseline function should be established with electrophysiological testing.

(b) Early surgical intervention is indicated.

(c) Most of the injuries are complete or partial transections.

(d) No evidence of recovery on clinical examination is an indication for surgery.

(e) Focal lesions should be explored at 2–3 months.

47. Myotoxicity:

    (a) LAs damage the whole of the muscle cell causing neurotoxicity.

    (b) Sarcoplasmic reticulum and mitochondria are the first organelles to be involved in injury.

    (c) Bupivacaine does not cause any toxicity.

    (d) Steroids if added to local anaesthetic prevents against muscle injury.

    (e) Extraocular muscles are resistant to damage by the local anaesthetics.

48. Opioid analgesics:

    (a) Brainstem rostral ventrolateral medulla is thought to be the main target for opioid respiratory depressant effect.

    (b) μ and κ receptors mediate the effects of opioids on bowel.

    (c) Laxatives should be prescribed for bowel ileus.

    (d) Cross-tolerance is seen with alcohol.

    (e) PCA is more effective in pain management in drug abusers.

49. Opioid-related complications:

    (a) Meperidine is most commonly involved with delirium.

    (b) Morphine metabolites are not active.

    (c) Morphine-6-glucronide accounts for dry mouth seen with use of opioids.

    (d) Respiratory depression is a κ-mediated effect.

    (e) Hypohydrosis is a common side effect.

50. Opioid-induced hypogonadism:
    (a) Depression may be a presenting feature of hypogonadism.
    (b) Is seen due to peripheral inhibition of gonadotrophins.
    (c) Methadone does not cause hypogonadotropic effects.
    (d) Reduced bone density can be seen in association with hypogonadotropism.
    (e) Side effect of testosterone treatment is sleep apnoea.

Answers

1. (a) T   (b) T   (c) T   (d) T   (e) T

   Quality is better than systemically administered analgesics. Analgesia up to 12 h is possible with 0.5 % bupivacaine for limb surgery. Insertion of catheter can increase the duration of block for few days. In patients with diabetes, poor pain management can destabilise the insulin requirements which are further worsened by opioid usage. Improved graft survival is seen because of sympathectomy. Better outcomes are seen in plastic and reconstructive surgery.

2. (a) T   (b) T   (c) T   (d) T   (e) T

   Davis et al. showed that spinal anaesthesia decreased blood loss during hip replacement surgery. Christopher et al. showed that compared with general anaesthesia, epidural anaesthesia is associated with a lower incidence of reoperation for inadequate tissue perfusion and therefore main be advantageous for this surgical population. The paper showed 50 % reduction in the overall incidence of shivering in patients who received fentanyl, and there was some evidence to suggest that low-dose epidural fentanyl might reduce shivering by an influence on thermoregulation. Epidural analgesia with bupivacaine and morphine provided the best balance of analgesia and side effects while accelerating post-operative recovery of gastrointestinal function and time to fulfilment of discharge criteria in relatively healthy patients. The presence of epidural analgesia was associated with a significantly lower odds of death at 7 days.

3. (a) T   (b) F   (c) F   (d) T   (e) F

4. (a) F   (b) F   (c) T   (d) T   (e) T

5. (a) T   (b) T   (c) F   (d) F   (e) F

The overall metabolic effect of the hormonal changes is increased catabolism which mobilises substrates to provide energy sources and a mechanism to retain salt and water and maintain fluid volume and cardiovascular hemostasis. Both skeletal muscle protein and visceral protein get broken down.

6. (a) T   (b) T   (c) T   (d) F   (e) T

Elimination of ileus allows early use of enteral nutrition which is an important factor in reducing the risk of infectious complications. Regional analgesic techniques reduce the incidence of thromboembolic complications following surgery of the pelvis and lower limbs. In upper abdominal procedures, there is not quite the same benefit in the incidence of thrombotic episodes.

7. (a) F   (b) T   (c) T   (d) T   (e) T

Only growth hormone and prolactin are increased in response to a surgical stimulus. A feedback mechanism operates so that increased concentrations of circulating cortisol inhibit further secretions of ACTH. This control mechanism appears to be ineffective after surgery so that concentrations of both hormones remain high. Growth hormone stimulates protein synthesis, promotes lipolysis and has an anti-insulin effect.

8. (a) T   (b) F   (c) T   (d) F   (e) F

Prolactin decrease is seen only with regional anaesthesia as general anaesthesia has a stimulatory effect on prolactin. Hyperglycaemic response is blocked by inhibition of hepatic glycogenolytic response to surgery. Post-operative oxygen consumption is decreased because of inhibitory catecholamine response to surgery.

9. (a) T   (b) F   (c) T   (d) F   (e) T

10. (a) T   (b) F   (c) T   (d) F

Verbal consent is admissible, but a note should be made in the notes. Only complications >1 % should be mentioned. Informed consent, proper disclosure, effective communication and an appropriate ethical approach can prevent legal complications.

11. (a) T   (b) T   (c) T   (d) T   (e) T

All complications should be discussed including convulsions, cardiac toxicity, nerve injury and awareness during conscious sedation. Some patients are not psychologically stable for regional anaesthesia (e.g. schizophrenia, anatomical distortion, fixed cardiac outputs).

12. (a) T   (b) T   (c) T   (d) T   (e) F

INR > 2 is a relative contraindication for ophthalmic anaesthesia.

13. (a) T   (b) F   (c) T   (d) T   (e) T

Pulse oximetry is also required as a standard recommended by ASA and the association of anaesthetists of Great Britain and Ireland.

14. (a) F   (b) T   (c) F   (d) T   (e) T

A single dose of warfarin results in prolongation of prothrombin time in approximately 20 % of patients. Enhanced sensitivity to warfarin is seen in females, age >65, excessive surgical blood loss, liver or renal disease. Fondaparinux is a synthetic pentasaccharide which produces its antithrombotic effect by inhibiting factor Xa and has a half-life of 20 h which allows once a day dosage.

15. (a) T   (b) F   (c) T   (d) T   (e) T

Sympathetic effects seen are decrease in heart rate, systolic blood pressure, stroke volume and cardiac output. Pulmonary function is improved because of profound analgesia.

16. (a) T   (b) F   (c) T   (d) T   (e) F

The incidence of spinal hematoma is 1 in 150,000 epidural and less than 1 in 220,000 spinal anaesthetics. Most hematomas become symptomatic several days after needle/catheter placement. Other risk factors are anticoagulant effect, increased age, female gender, history of gastrointestinal bleeding, aspirin use and length of therapy. The incidence of haemorrhagic complications with heparin is <3 % and with thrombolytic therapy is between 6 and 30 %.

17. (a) T   (b) F   (c) T   (d) T   (e) F

Most common injury seen is neuropraxia. Mostly, the healing is seen within 3 months which is the amount of time required for axonal regeneration.

18. (a) T   (b) F   (c) T   (d) T   (e) T

Blunt needles are more disruptive than sharp needles. The pressure of injection should be less than 20 psi.

19. (a) T (b) T (c) T (d) T (e) T

Brown-Sequard syndrome is characterised by loss of motor function, loss of vibration sense and fine touch, loss of proprioception, and loss of two point discrimination and signs of weakness on the same side of body. Patient positioning is important for nerve injury, e.g. peroneal nerve at fibular head and brachial plexus because of hypertension during thoracotomy.

20. (a) T (b) F (c) F (d) T (e) T

The incidence with interscalene block is 3 % whereas the incidence with supraclavicular varies from 6 to 23 %. Right side is more common because cupola on right side is higher. Chest drain is required if degree of lung collapse is >25 %. Risk is reduced in vertical techniques because the needle is not directed toward the lung.

21. (a) T (b) T (c) F (d) T (e) T

It is frequently seen with supraclavicular technique.

22. (a) T (b) F (c) T (d) T (e) T

It is motor to diaphragm with sensory innervations to pleura, mediastinum and upper abdomen. Permanent palsy is seen but is rare. There is an associated 27 % decrease in FVC and 26 % decrease in FEV.

23. (a) T (b) T (c) T (d) T (e) F

Patient with right to left shunts does not have uptake of drugs by lungs which sequester up to 80 % of intravenous medication. This increases the likelihood of CNS toxicity. Sick sinus syndrome is associated with automaticity of lower pacemakers and conduction disturbances. Local anaesthetics that diminish sino-atrial node activity, increase the cardiac refractory period, prolong the intracardiac conduction time and lengthen the QRS complex will aggravate sinus node dysfunction. Epidural injection at or above T4 level delays gastric emptying. This can contribute to gastric regurgitation and aspiration along with the palsy of recurrent laryngeal nerve, a complication of blockades in the neck region. Glucose-6-phosphate dehydrogenase deficiency can cause methemoglobinemia with benzocaine, lidocaine and prilocaine. Although it has been stated that neither amide nor ester-linked local anaesthetics are contraindicated in such cases, any drug that releases calcium from sarcoplasm reticulum, such as lidocaine, should be avoided.

24. (a) T   (b) F   (c) T   (d) T   (e) T

The onset can be immediate. Axial length >26 mm is a risk factor along with retinal detachment, those who require refractive surgery.

25. (a) T   (b) F   (c) F   (d) T   (e) T

Heparin at a dosage of 5,000 units requires 1-h gap after insertion or removal of catheter. Heparin-induced thrombocytopenia is a risk for those getting infusions for more than 4 days, so monitoring should be started after 4 days.

26. (a) T   (b) T   (c) T   (d) T   (e) T

27. (a) T   (b) F   (c) T   (d) T

28. (a) T   (b) T   (c) F   (d) T   (e) F

Risk of toxicity in peripheral system is increased in chronic renal failure due to increased blood flow due to hyperdynamic circulation in uraemia.

29. (a) T   (b) T   (c) T   (d) F   (e) F

Acid glycoprotein is elevated in chronic renal failure because of chronic inflammatory state because of altered cytokine secretion. Onset time is decreased because of volume contraction in intrathecal space. There is platelet dysfunction and impaired platelet vessel wall interaction, but there is higher prevalence of thrombotic events. There is toxic effect on binding of fibrinogen to platelet glycoprotein IIb/IIIa receptors. Highest arteriovenous blood flow with least hemodynamic changes are obtained with brachial plexus block than general anaesthesia.

30. (a) T   (b) F   (c) T   (d) F   (e) T

Amide anaesthetic toxicity is increased because of decrease in microsomal function, by which they are metabolised. In liver disease, both measured volume of distribution and plasma clearance are reduced; therefore, the drug dosages should be decreased because of low clearance. Grape juice can inhibit microsomal enzyme and increase toxicity. High epidural block (T1–T4) is associated with decreased hepatic blood flow because of effect on splanchnic circulation.

31. (a) T   (b) F   (c) T   (d) T   (e) T

There is a higher risk of ischaemia in diabetes mellitus because of pre-existing neuropathy. Location by nerve stimulator is not reliable in diabetes because of associated decreased conduction velocity and amplitude of both motor and sensory nerves. Double crush syndrome is increased susceptibility of nerves to injury or impairment at one anatomic location, when already compressed or otherwise injured at another location.

32. (a) F   (b) F   (c) T   (d) F   (e) F

Factor 7 has the shortest life (6–8 h). INR may be normal with concomitant decrease in factors II and X. PT and INR are most sensitive to activities of factor VII and insensitive to factor II. INR > 1.2 is seen when factor VII is reduced to approximately 55 % of baseline. INR = 1.5 when factor VII activity decreases to approximately 40 % of normal. As normal hemostasis requires 40 % of factor activity, normal hemostasis can be achieved with INR < 1.5. Garlic is a herbal medication which inhibits platelet aggregation and increases fibrinolysis.

Factor	Half-life (h)
Factor VII	6–8
Factor IX	24
Factor X	25–60
Factor II	50–80

33. (a) T   (b) F   (c) T   (d) T   (e) T

Ticlodipine and clopidogrel interfere with platelet fibrinogen binding and subsequent platelet-platelet interactions and lasts for the life of platelets. Clopidogrel needs to be stopped for 5 days, while ticlodipine warrants stoppage for 14 days. Abciximab, eptifibatide and tirofiban belong to glycoprotein IIb/IIIa receptor antagonists and inhibit platelet aggregation by interfering with platelet fibrinogen binding. Ginko is a herbal medication with duration of action of 36 h.

34. (a) F   (b) F   (c) F   (d) T   (e) F

Staphylococcus aureus is seen in more than 50 % of patients having epidural abscess. The frequency of epidural infection is 1–2/10,000 hospital admissions as compared to frequency of intravenous catheter-related infections which are 1:50,000. Steroid administration adversely affects the outcome. The risk factors associated are prolonged catheter in situ, being immunocompromised and being critically ill. Surgery within 12 h is associated with best chances of recovery.

35. (a) T   (b) F   (c) T   (d) F   (e) T

Lidocaine and bupivacaine have shown bacteriostatic qualities, but *S. aureus* and coagulase-negative *Staphylococcus* are inhibited at concentrations greater than 2 % lidocaine and 0.5 % bupivacaine. Catheter hub infections account for more than 50 % of infections. Infections have been seen even after the use of filter as antimicrobial effectiveness decreases with prolonged usage.

36. (a) T   (b) T   (c) F

Incidence is 61 %. Other risk factors involved are admission to ICU, male gender, catheter insertion more than 48 h and lack of antibiotic prophylaxis.

37. (a) T   (b) F   (c) T   (d) T   (e) T

Clonidine is an alpha 2 agonist. It also causes hypotension by decreasing heart rate, by presynaptic inhibition of norepinephrine increase and by direct parasympathetic effect. Stimulation of Bezold–Jarisch reflex increases parasympathetic activity and decrease sympathetic activity. Poorly filled ventricle (caused by upright posture) and vigorous myocardial contractility can contribute. Interscalene block can cause a decrease in left ventricular volume in sitting position and enhances cardiac contractility because of addition of epinephrine to local anaesthetic.

38. (a) T   (b) T   (c) F   (d) F   (e) F

The risk is more in hip surgery because of occurrence of embolic material migrating to heart and lungs during cement hip arthroplasty, causing acute pulmonary embolism-type hemodynamic response. Low cardiac output occurs secondary to right heart distension causing failure leading to bradycardia and cardiac arrest. Prehydration has been seen to cause significant reduction in incidence of hypotension but only for a short time. The arrests seen are primarily non-hypoxic.

39. (a) T   (b) T   (c) F   (d) F   (e) T

R isomer is 1.5 times to 2.5 times more toxic than S isomer. cAMP production is decreased due to inhibition at the beta-receptors or at adenyl cyclise level. Bupivacaine is more potent at producing arrythemias. True allergy is rare with amides but seen more commonly with ester local anaesthetics that are metabolised directly to para-aminobenzoic acid.

40. (a) T   (b) T   (c) F   (d) F   (e) T

Other signs of toxicity are tinnitus, confusion, restlessness, perioral tingling, metallic taste and sense of impending doom. Both metabolic and respiratory acidosis decrease convulsive dose. CC/CNS ratio: dose that produces cardiotoxicity to dose that produces CNS toxicity (CC/CNS ratio—bupivacaine < levobupivacaine < ropivacaine).

41. (a) T   (b) T   (c) F   (d) T   (e) T

Local anaesthetics and epinephrine significantly reduce peripheral nerve blood flow. Low-dosage epidural usage results in uptake and decreases systemic vascular resistance and increases cardiac output.

42. (a) T   (b) F   (c) T   (d) T   (e) T

Clonidine is an alpha 2 agonist that binds to receptors in substantia gelatinosa and the intermediolateral cell column. The neurophysiologic consequence is to inhibit release of substance P and firing of wide dynamic range neurons in dorsal horn. Neostigmine prevents breakdown of acetylcholine in dorsal horn, with effects at the muscarinic receptors in substantia gelatinosa, thought to result in analgesia. Ketamine is a phencyclidine-related analgesic that binds at gated calcium channels of the NMDA receptors, producing a non-competitive blockade. Magnesium is a non-competitive antagonist at NMDA receptors. Midazolam is a water-soluble benzodiazepine.

43. (a) F   (b) F   (c) T   (d) F   (e) F

Transient neurologic symptoms is the term used to describe both unilateral or bilateral pain occurring within 24 h after spinal anaesthesia that involves buttocks and may radiate to lower extremities. Symptoms begin within 24 h after the resolution of spinal anaesthesia. Pain is mostly unilateral or bilateral, mostly in the buttocks. Symptoms can take 6 h to 4 days to resolve. There are no neurological findings on physical examination or imaging. There is significant impairment of daily functional activities like walking, sitting and sleeping.

44. (a) F   (b) T   (c) T   (d) T   (e) F

In Wallerian degeneration, components distal to the site of injury will degenerate and be destroyed by phagocytosis. It takes about 4 weeks to finish. Primary or retrograde degeneration occurs primarily and proceeds for at least one intermodal space. Severe injury may be evident by chromatolysis (swelling of cytoplasm with eccentric displacement of cell's nucleus). Nissl substance is rough endoplasmic reticulum and a site of protein synthesis. Axonal regeneration starts within 24 h.

45. (a) F   (b) F   (c) T   (d) T   (e) T

Double crush injury: patients with pre-existing neurologic deficits may be more susceptible to injury at another site, when exposed to a secondary insult. The second insult need not be along the peripheral nerve trunk but rather at any point along the nerve transmission pathway.

Known surgical factors include: intraoperative trauma, vascular compromise, perioperative infection, hematoma formation, tourniquet ischaemia and improperly applied casts. Direct surgical trauma is seen in 40 % of patients.

46. (a) T   (b) F   (c) F   (d) F   (e) T

Most of the injuries are neuropraxias, and electrophysiologic testing should be done to ascertain baseline function. Most of the times, conservative measures (limb protection, physical rehabilitation, range of motion exercises) are effective. The vast majority of injuries are transient and self-limited neuropraxias. Patients with persistent (6–8 weeks) symptoms of progressive neurologic deficit should undergo neurosurgical evaluation.

47. (a) F   (b) T   (c) F   (d) F   (e) T

Myotoxicity is seen with local anaesthetics because of direct action of local anaesthetics on the muscle cell (myocyte) that initiates a cellular process leading to destruction of the cell. Only adult myocytes are damaged; basal laminae, vasculature, neural elements and immature myocytes remain intact and thus account for regeneration in 3–4 weeks. Early changes are seen in organelles with changes in sarcoplasmic reticulum and mitochondria seen as early as 15 min. Bupivacaine produces most intense myonecrosis and procaine the least. The risk factors for myotoxicity are high dosage, direct intramuscular injection and addition of adjuvants like adrenaline and steroids. Extraocular muscles have more mitochondria and may explain the lower sensitivity of extraocular muscles to local anaesthetics compared with other somatic muscles.

48. (a) T   (b) T   (c) F   (d) T   (e) T

Respiratory depression is a well-known effect of opioids. Rostral ventrolateral medulla is chief generator of respiratory rhythm, and depression can be seen with opioids. μ and κ receptors, present in gut's myenteric plexus, increase the tone of bowel luminal musculature and stimulating sphincters leading to delayed transit time for contents and increased time for fluid absorption. Constipation is seen with chronic opioid use, and if untreated it causes faecal impaction. Ileus tends to occur in surgical patients, or after trauma, and opioids prolong ileus. Ileus usually responds to normal feeding. Patient-controlled analgesia provides an element of control and lessens anxiety associated with trying to obtain additional medication.

49. (a) T   (b) F   (c) T   (d) F   (e) F

Meperidine's main metabolite is normeperidine. It causes neurotoxicity especially in elderly patients and those with poor renal function. Morphine-3-glucronide and morphine-6-glucronide are two major water-soluble morphine metabolites dependant on renal elimination. Morphine-3-glucronide has antinociceptive properties and is associated with hyperalgesia and myoclonus. Morphine-6-glucronide is a potent analgesic and may be more potent than morphine. Respiratory depression is a μ receptor-mediated effect in brain stem. Hyperhidrosis is a common side effect and is thought to be related to mast cell degranulation and is controlled with antihistaminics.

50. (a) T   (b) F   (c) F   (d) T   (e) T

Symptoms of hypogonadism seen are loss of libido, impotence, infertility, depression, anxiety, fatigue, loss of muscle mass and strength. Opioids bind to receptors in hypothalamus, pituitary and testes to modulate gonadal function. Opioids also have a direct inhibitory effect on the testes to decrease production of testosterone. Similar effects are seen with methadone causing decrease of testosterone which is observed as soon as within 4 h of administration. Common side effects of testosterone are local site reaction, sleep apnoea and polycythemia.

2 Equipment and Usage of Ultrasound

1. Peripheral nerve stimulation:
   (a) Rely on use of electric current to elicit motor stimulation.
   (b) Depolarisation can result both in contraction of effector muscles and paraesthesias.
   (c) Same principle can be used for percutaneous guidance and epidural catheter placement.
   (d) Rise of high-intensity stimulating current with a short pulse width can prevent uncomfortable motor response to nerve stimulation.
   (e) Limiting energy or current intensity can avoid discomfort.

2. The quality of stimulation of peripheral nerves depend on:
   (a) Polarity of electrode
   (b) Distance between stimulating needle and nerve
   (c) Interaction at the tissue-needle interface
   (d) Type of electrode
   (e) Frequency of stimulus

3. Intensity of nerve stimulation:
   (a) Total charge applied = intensity of applied current × duration of square pulse of current.
   (b) Rheobase is the minimum current density required to repolarise the nerve.
   (c) Chronaxie is the minimum duration of pulse required to depolarise the nerve.

R. Gupta, D. Patel, *Multiple Choice Questions in Regional Anaesthesia*,
DOI 10.1007/978-3-642-31257-1_2, © Springer-Verlag Berlin Heidelberg 2013

(d) The shorter the fibre, the easier is it to stimulate.
(e) Myelinated fibres require less electrical energy for activation.

4. Stimulation of nerve fibres:
    (a) Rectangular pulses are used.
    (b) Membrane time constant determines properties of the cell.
    (c) Normal membrane time constant is 10 ms.
    (d) Nerve fibres get easily stimulated when anode is applied to them.
    (e) Frequency and pulse duration are the main parameters influencing stimulation of nerves.

5. Coulomb's law:
    (a) Reflects that stimulation intensity is variable.
    (b) $E = k(q/r^2)$.
    (c) Values >8 are safe.
    (d) Electrical resistance of human body for wet skin is 10 KΩ.
    (e) Resistance of energy source is not important.

6. Peripheral nerve stimulation:
    (a) Negative electrode is cathode and positive electrode is anode.
    (b) Final intensity of current should be less than 0.3 mA to ensure a high success rate.
    (c) If motor-evoked activity disappears after injecting 1–2 ml, needle repositioning is required.
    (d) PNS technique reduces latency time but prolongs performance time.
    (e) Insulated needles give less satisfactory results than non-insulated ones.

7. Peripheral nerve stimulus:
    (a) Depends on both sensory and motor responses.
    (b) Direct muscle stimulation can give a false stimulating sign.
    (c) Metameric response is seen with stimulation of trunks.
    (d) Median nerve stimulation produces palm flexion and opposition of thumb.
    (e) Radial nerve stimulation causes extension of elbow and or wrist.

8. Advantages of peripheral nerve stimulation:
    (a) Increases the success rate of technique
    (b) Decreases the requirements of local anaesthetic
    (c) Helps in developing new approaches
    (d) Easy availability
    (e) Fewer injections required for block

9. Needles for regional anaesthesia:
    (a) Standard shaft length is 8 cm.
    (b) Whitacre needles have large side opening hole.
    (c) Tuohy, Crawford and husted needles are used for spinal anaesthesia.
    (d) The side port in pencil-point needle is designed to prevent intraneural injection.
    (e) Bevel angle is determined by British standards.

10. Ideal characteristics of peripheral nerve stimulator:
    (a) Portable battery operated, with detachable and sterilised needles
    (b) Should have clear markings for attachment to cathode
    (c) Short duration impulse so that sensory nerves are preferentially stimulated

  (d) Sensitivity should not be allowed to fall <1 mA
  (e) Universal terminal for use with variety
       of needles

11. Equipment for regional anaesthesia:
  (a) Standard notation for needles is size of external
       diameter.
  (b) Two factors determining needle diameter are
       viscosity of fluid and rigidity required for insertion.
  (c) Catheters are usually made of reactive material so
       that fibrosis consolidates their position.
  (d) Filters should block everything less than
       0.22 µm.
  (e) All catheters have single terminal opening.

12. Spinal needle:
  (a) Main consideration in design is a need to minimise
       PDPH.
  (b) Quincke's needle has a blunt tip.
  (c) Stillete should be in place while inserting the
       needle.
  (d) Micro spinal catheters can cause cauda equina
       syndrome.
  (e) Identification of back flow of CSF is easy with 29 G
       needle.

13. Following are true about epidural needle:
  (a) Internal diameter should be large enough to allow a
       suitable-sized catheter.
  (b) External diameter should be as small as possible to
       allow ease of insertion.
  (c) The catheter should not buckle while
       insertion.
  (d) 16–18 G can be used for children.
  (e) The Huber tip has an angle of 45°.

14. Epidural catheter markings:
    (a) Double markings at the tip
    (b) Five single markings 1 cm apart
    (c) Double markings at 15 cm
    (d) Quadruple markings at 20 cm
    (e) No markings between 11 and 14 cm

15. Peripheral nerve block needles:
    (a) Short bevelled needles allow user to feel fascial planes more easily.
    (b) Sprotte needle allows passage of catheter parallel to the nerve.
    (c) Tuohy needle with Huber tip can be used for placing catheters.
    (d) Failure rate is decreased by using insulated needles.
    (e) Desirable quality is separate injection port in the side arm.

16. Peripheral nerve block catheters:
    (a) Multiple side-hole catheters are best suited for block.
    (b) Removable wire stiffeners make passage between fascial planes easier.
    (c) Can be made radiopaque.
    (d) Stimulating catheters help reduce the problem of secondary block failure.
    (e) Stimulating catheters have metallic spiral in its wall.

17. Peripheral nerve stimulation:
    (a) Accommodation is best prevented by using a square wave of current with a sharp rising time.
    (b) Anode site is not critical when using a constant current output nerve stimulator.
    (c) The threshold current relation is inverse of square of the distance.

   (d) Relation between current intensity and distance is governed by Coulomb's law.
   (e) The most common acceptable current range with a clear motor response is 0.2–0.5 mA.

18. Advantages of ultrasound:
   (a) Reveals anatomical details.
   (b) Real time imaging guidance during needle advancement.
   (c) Local anaesthetic spread is not visible.
   (d) Improves quality of sensory block, onset time and success rate compared to nerve stimulation techniques.
   (e) Decrease the number of needle attempts.

19. Ultrasound:
   (a) Frequency is >20,000 Hz.
   (b) Falls within human hearing range.
   (c) A wave is generated as electric field is applied to piezoelectric crystal.
   (d) Waves of large pulse lengths improve axial resolution.
   (e) Pulse radio frequency should be between 1 and 10 KHz.

20. Ultrasound image:
   (a) Is due to piezoelectric effect.
   (b) Transducer is required to apply high-amplitude voltage to energise the crystals.
   (c) Attenuation is due to absorption only.
   (d) Bone has a high attenuation coefficient.
   (e) Attenuation is independent of frequency.

21. Attenuation seen in imaging:
   (a) Water has highest attenuation coefficient.
   (b) Gain is the amplification achieved.

(c) Air has lowest acoustic impedance.
(d) The higher the degree of impedance mismatch, the greater the amount of reflection.
(e) Attenuation also results from reflection and scattering.

22. Artefacts of ultrasound:
   (a) Specular reflection occurs at rough surfaces.
   (b) Wavelength of ultrasound wave must be greater than reflective structure to cause specular reflection.
   (c) Scattering is seen in visceral organs.
   (d) Refraction occurs when speed of sound is different on each side of tissue interface.
   (e) Bone causes maximum refraction.

23. Echogenicity:
   (a) Strong specular reflections produce hypoechoic shadows.
   (b) Solid organs are hypoechoic.
   (c) Fluid and blood appears dark.
   (d) Deep structures are hyperechoic.
   (e) Muscles have heterogenous appearance.

24. Tissue echogenicity:
   (a) Vein and arteries both are collapsible.
   (b) Bone has a hyperechoic outline and hypoechoic bony shadow underneath.
   (c) Muscle has highly hyperechoic outline.
   (d) Degree of hypergenicity likely reflects the amount of connective tissue within the nerve.
   (e) There is a change of echogenicity of tissues as a result of transducer angle.

25. Image resolution:
    (a) Is the ability of ultrasound to distinguish two structures that are close together as separate.
    (b) A high-frequency wave with a short pulse length will yield better axial resolution than a low-frequency wave.
    (c) A high-frequency transducer emits a wave with a short wavelength.
    (d) Attenuation decreases with increase in frequency.
    (e) Both axial and lateral resolutions are important.

26. Doppler:
    (a) A moving source and a stationary listener are required.
    (b) Source moving away from receiver will give red shadow.
    (c) Detection of flow is best when transducer is perpendicular to vessel.
    (d) Colour power Doppler can distinguish vascular from non-vascular structures.
    (e) CPD is more sensitive than colour Doppler in flow direction.

27. Power Doppler:
    (a) Is based on estimating the integrated Doppler power spectrum.
    (b) More sensitive at detecting blood flow.
    (c) The signal is dependent on the angle between the vessel and the transducer beam.
    (d) Artefacts are not seen.
    (e) There are no disadvantages.

28. Image artefacts:
    (a) Acoustic enhancement artefact is seen deep to a fluid-filled structure.
    (b) Tissue reverberation artefact is seen when beam meets bone.

(c) Lung tissue gives specular reflection.
(d) Reverberation artefacts are seen during needle advancement.
(e) Large dropout artefact is seen in air artefact.

29. Needle visibility:
    (a) Main factors determining ultrasonic visibility of needle is insertion angle and gauge of the needle.
    (b) Needle tip visibility is decreased at steep angle.
    (c) Large bore needles are easy to see as they are less likely to bend.
    (d) A dark background enhances tip visibility.
    (e) In-plane techniques prevent vascular punctures.

30. Needle tip visibility:
    (a) Is best seen when beam angles perpendicular to the needle.
    (b) Mean brightness has a linear correlation with angle of incidence.
    (c) Spatial compound imaging improves the needle tip imaging.
    (d) Bevel direction has no effect on tip visualisation.
    (e) Increasing needle diameter improves visualisation of needle tip.

31. Nerve Imaging:
    (a) Cervical nerve roots have mono-fascicular appearance.
    (b) Most peripheral nerves have mono-fascicular appearance.
    (c) Short-axis scanning is better to scan the course of nerve.
    (d) Tendons have similar appearance to nerve.
    (e) Tendons are more anisotropic than nerves.

32. Nerve identification:
    (a) Peripheral nerves have a honeycomb appearance.
    (b) The best way to follow a nerve is by use of linear transducer.
    (c) Long-axis views are the preferred method of nerve visualisation.
    (d) Nerves as small as 1 mm in diameter can be visualised.
    (e) Dynamic ultrasound imaging is best seen with popliteal fossa.

33. Local anaesthetic injection:
    (a) Agitated solutions are best to visualise nerve.
    (b) Bubbles can disperse in tissue and cause acoustic shadowing.
    (c) Bicarbonate-containing solutions of local anaesthetic helps in clarity of image.
    (d) Needle should touch the nerve while injecting solution so as to cause maximum effect.
    (e) Unagitated solution outlines the borders of anaesthetised nerve.

34. Short-axis imaging of nerves:
    (a) Identification of peripheral nerves is easy on short axis.
    (b) Resolution of fascial barriers around nerves is not good.
    (c) Circumferential distribution of local anaesthetic can be seen.
    (d) More mobility of transducer is possible.

35. Ultrasound imaging in tissues:
    (a) Specular reflection is seen with smooth surface.
    (b) Scattering reflection is seen with smooth surface.
    (c) Most neutral images are seen with specular reflection.
    (d) Acoustic impedance of tissue surrounding nerve is not important.

    (e) Most neural images are seen with specular reflection.

    (f) Best view is seen if needle is parallel to ultrasound beam.

36. Attenuation:
    (a) Progressive loss of acoustic energy as a wave passes through tissue.
    (b) Absorption is the main source of ultrasound attenuation.
    (c) It is measured in db/mm of tissue.
    (d) Time gain compensation can help in offsetting effects of attenuation.
    (e) The higher the attenuation coefficient, the more attenuated the ultrasound waves.

37. Resolution of ultrasound:
    (a) Ability of ultrasound to distinguish one object from another.
    (b) Axial resolution is the ability to separate two structures lying at different depths.
    (c) Lower frequency produces best axial resolution.
    (d) Lower frequency probes allow for deeper tissue penetration.
    (e) Higher frequency transducer probes effect high axial resolution of superficial structures.

38. Contact artefact:
    (a) Seen when there is loss of acoustic coupling between transducer and skin.
    (b) Can be minimised by application of gel.
    (c) Air bubbles trapped in gel can contribute to contact artefact.
    (d) Needle insertion close to transducer helps in avoiding the artefact.
    (e) Firm pressure with transducer is required for optimal block.

39. Anisotropy:
    (a) Amplitude of received echoes varies with angle of insonation.
    (b) With nerves, angle changes as small as 10° from axis can decrease echogenicity.
    (c) Angle changes have no effect on anisotropy on tendons.
    (d) Anisotropy is seen more with tendons than nerves.

40. Needle tip visibility:
    (a) Strong specular reflections occur from beam angle perpendicular to the needle.
    (b) Linear correlation between angle of incidence and mean brightness.
    (c) Beam steering to different angles helps visualise needle tip.
    (d) Needle tip is best visualised when bevel is oriented either directly towards or away from transducer.
    (e) Needle visualisation is better for superficial blocks.

41. Ultrasound image:
    (a) Gain allows operator to change brightness of image.
    (b) Time gain compensation allows operator to adjust the brightness independently at specific depths in the field.
    (c) Temporal resolution is important for visualising moving objects.
    (d) Temporal resolution is improved by adjusting focus.
    (e) Ultrasound beam first converges to a point and then diverges.

42. Acoustic artefacts:
    (a) Both missing structures and degraded images can contribute to this.
    (b) Only overgain is associated with artefacts.

(c) Acoustic shadowing is mostly seen in structures lying deep to bone.

(d) Calcified arterial plaques can cause acoustic shadowing.

(e) Acoustic enhancement is seen in infraclavicular and axillary brachial plexus.

43. Reverberation artefact:

(a) Occur as a result of ultrasound waves bouncing between two specular reflectors

(b) Seen more if needle is parallel to ultrasound beam

(c) Multiple reverberation artefacts can merge to increase image disturbance.

(d) Needle may actually appear deeper than it is because of the artefact.

(e) Increase gain can help decrease reverberation artefact.

44. Coulomb's law:

(a) $E = K(Q/R^2)$

(b) Motor response at low amperage means nerve is close to electrode.

(c) Decrease in amperage leads to increased sensitivity.

(d) Higher current density is associated with patient discomfort.

(e) Defibrillation pods have high resistance.

45. Electrical pulse duration:

(a) Duration of periodic pulse square wave generated by nerve stimulation.

(b) Typically long pulse durations are used for nerve localisation.

(c) Increased duration increases severity of localisation.

(d) Decreased duration increases specificity of localisation.

(e) Increased pulse duration increases total flow of electrons.

46. Percutaneous electrode stimulation:
    (a) Coupling gel is not required.
    (b) Indentation of skin with stimulation probe facilitates nerve stimulation.
    (c) Pure sensory nerves cannot be localised.
    (d) Normally not possible to stimulate C78T1.
    (e) Stimulation of phrenic nerve means electrode is anterior to plexus.

47. Multiple injection techniques:
    (a) Individual nerves are localised and blocked.
    (b) Evidence shows multiple injections better than single injection.
    (c) Allows reduction in the volume of local anaesthetic solution.
    (d) Only helpful in upper limb injections.
    (e) Multiple injections may delay onset of block.

48. Ultrasound guidance in children:
    (a) 5–10-MHz transducer is used.
    (b) Most reliable way is to insert it transversely.
    (c) Precise location of needle tip on ultrasound image is a prerequisite for effective block.
    (d) Children are more at risk for local anaesthetic toxicity than adults.
    (e) Peripheral nerves are visualised with linear transducers.

49. Ultrasound in neuraxial block:
    (a) Is as good as physical examination for identifying the level.
    (b) Ligamentum flavum is hypoechoic on ultrasound.
    (c) Cerebrospinal fluid is hyperechoic.
    (d) Can help in determining the depth of needle penetration.
    (e) Paramedian region is better for ultrasound visualisation.

50. Stimulating catheters:
    (a) The electrically conducting connection extends to proximal 5 cm of catheter only.
    (b) 14-gauge needle is required to insert catheter.
    (c) Once the catheter is in position, saline should be injected to expand space.
    (d) Both sensory and motor stimulation can be achieved with stimulating catheters.
    (e) Long-term infusions require special catheter securing techniques.

Answers

1. (a) T   (b) T   (c) T   (d) F   (e) T

    A weak current is applied to stimulating needle with the help of a current generator (nerve stimulator) to elicit motor stimulation. Low intensity with short pulse width can avoid motor response. Same principal applies for transcutaneous stimulation though longer pulse duration is required.

2. (a) T   (b) T   (c) T   (d) T   (e) T

    Less electrical energy is required if cathode (−ve) is close to the nerve. Anodal stimulation requires a higher current to stimulate the nerve. Distance is governed by Coulomb's law:

    $$I = K(q / y^2)^2$$

    I = current required to stimulate nerve, K = constant, Q = minimal current for stimulation and V = the distance from stimulus to nerve.

    If frequency is low, nerve may be penetrated. If frequency is high, painful muscles may be induced.

3. (a) T   (b) F   (c) T   (d) F   (e) T

    Rheobase: It is the minimum current required to depolarise the nerve. Chronaxie: the stimulus duration needed for impulse generation when employing a current strength twice the rheobase. The larger the fibre, the shorter is the chronaxie and easier to stimulate. Similarly, myelinated fibres are much more sensitive and require less energy for stimulation than unmyelinated fibres (chronaxie of α fibres-50-100; δ-170; c-400).

4. (a) T   (b) T   (c) T   (d) F   (e) T

A rectangular pulse helps avoid prolonged currents. Membrane time constant represents the time that it takes to change the membrane capacitance. At anode, displacement of positive charge towards exterior of membrane increases the voltage across it. This produces a state of hyperpolarisation that diminishes excitability. Ideal frequency is 1–2 Hz and pulse duration is 1–2 ms.

5. (a) T   (b) T   (c) F   (d) T   (e) F

Values greater than 8 would require such significant strength stimuli that systemic side effects may result. The resistance between surface electrodes is 25 KΩ, and with penetration of dermis, it comes down to 0.5 KΩ. The internal resistance should always be greater than that of human body (1 KΩ).

6. (a) T   (b) F   (c) F   (d) T   (e) F

Cathode is attached to machine and anode to patient as neutral return electrode. Insulated needles give more precise location of nerve and require less current.

7. (a) F   (b) T   (c) T   (d) T   (e) T

8. (a) T   (b) T   (c) T   (d) T   (e) T

Peripheral nerve stimulator helps in developing new approaches like infraclavicular approach to brachial plexus. Less injections are required if PNS is used as in axillary block.

9. (a) T   (b) F   (c) F   (d) T   (e) T

Needle length variation is 25–100 mm for special needs. Sprotte needle has side opening hole. All three needles used for epidural injections.

10. (a) T   (b) T   (c) F   (d) F   (e) T

11. (a) T (b) T (c) F (d) T (e) F

Epidural needles are of 16 G and 18 G to minimise bending. Oil-based agents will pass through large diameter needles. Catheters are usually made of inert material so that they do not produce tissue reaction.

12. (a) T (b) F (c) T (d) T (e) F

Quincke's needle has a sharp cutting edge, while Whitacre and Sprotte have pencil-point and bullet-shaped needles, respectively. Stillete prevents coring of superficial tissue. Repeated exposure of nerve roots with micro spinal catheters can cause cauda equina syndrome.

13. (a) T (b) T (c) T (d) F (e) F

19 G is available for children. Huber tip is <20°.

14. (a) F (b) T (c) F (d) T (e) F

There is a single marking at the tip. Double markings are at 10 cm.

15. (a) T (b) T (c) T (d) T (e) T

16. (a) F (b) T (c) T (d) T (e) T

One or more holes of the catheter may lie outside the fascial plane in which nerve lies. Wire stiffeners make passage easier but may increase the failure rate. The increased efficacy of stimulating catheters is contentious.

17. (a) T (b) T (c) T (d) T (e) T

A prolonged subthreshold stimulus or slowly rising current may reduce nerve excitability by inactivating Na conduction before depolarisation reaches its threshold.

18. (a) T (b) T (c) F (d) T (e) T

19. (a) T   (b) F   (c) T   (d) F   (e) T

Ultrasound falls in the frequency range of 20–20,000 Hz. Conversion of electrical to mechanical energy is called converse piezoelectric effect. Wave of short wavelength improves axial resolution. Pulse rate frequency is rate of pulses emitted by the transducer.

20. (a) T   (b) F   (c) F   (d) T   (e) F

Piezoelectric effect is due to conversion of sound to electric energy. Pulsar is required to apply high-amplitude voltage. Attenuation is due to absorption, reflection and scattering. Attenuation coefficient is measured in db/cm of tissue. Bone has a high attenuation coefficient with absorption greater than 80 %. A high-frequency wave is associated with high attenuation thus limiting tissue penetration, where as a low-frequency wave is associated with low tissue attenuation and deep tissue penetration.

21. (a) F   (b) T   (c) T   (d) T   (e) T

Waters' attenuation coefficient is 0.002 and bone's is 5. Increased gain amplifies the returning signal and not transmitted signal. Attenuation is the resistance of a tissue to passage of ultrasound signal.

22. (a) F   (b) F   (c) T   (d) T   (e) T

Smooth surface is a flat surface where transmitted wave is reflected in a single direction; seen in fascial planes, diaphragm. Specular reflection is seen when wavelength of ultrasound is less than the reflective structure. Scattering is seen where surface is not smooth.

23. (a) F   (b) T   (c) T   (d) F   (e) T

Attenuation limits beam transmission to reach the structures. Muscles have hyperechoic outline with hypoechoic background.

24. (a) F (b) T (c) T (d) T (e) T

25. (a) T (b) T (c) T (d) F (e) T

A high-frequency transducer emits a wave with a short wavelength and small width. Lateral resolution is poor when the structures lying side by side are located within the same beam length. Axial resolution is ability to distinguish two structures that lie along long axis where as lateral resolution is resolution of objects lying side by side.

26. (a) T (b) F (c) F (d) T (e) T

Increased frequency is seen when source moves towards receiver and appears red. The frequency is decreased when the source moves away from receiver and appears blue. Colour flow Doppler does not indicate flow direction.

27. (a) T (b) T (c) F (d) T (e) F

Power Doppler is based on estimating the integrated Doppler power spectrum instead of mean Doppler frequency shift. It is more sensitive at detecting blood flow than velocity imaging. Integrated power Doppler is independent of angle between vessel and transducer beam. Disadvantages are high motion sensitivity and lack of directional information.

28. (a) T (b) F (c) T (d) T (e) T

Image artefacts are display distortions and errors that may adversely affect image interpretation. Acoustic enhancement artefact is seen because of beam penetration through an area of low attenuation coefficient to an area of higher attenuation coefficient. Acoustic shadow artefact is seen when beam meets bone.

29. (a) T (b) F (c) T (d) T (e) T

30. (a) T (b) T (c) T (d) F (e) T

    Spatial compound imaging is beam steering to different angles to produce overlapping scans that will form a composite image. The needle is best visualised $q =$ when the bevel is oriented directly towards or away from the transducer.

31. (a) T (b) T (c) T (d) T (e) F

32. (a) T (b) T (c) F (d) T (e) T

    Short-axis view gives appearance of honeycomb on peripheral nerves. Transverse scanning using a broad linear transducer is method of choice for following a nerve along its course. Though long-axis views are useful for panoramic views, they are time consuming and difficult to construct. Nerve motion can be revealed by dynamic ultrasound imaging and best seen in popliteal fossa where "seesaw" movement is seen with foot movement.

33. (a) F (b) T (c) F (d) F (e) T

    Agitated solution is best suited for visualising needle. Injection of small amount of air (0.3–0.5 ml) can be used to identify location of tip. Bicarbonate-containing solutions evolve CO_2 obscuring image.

34. (a) T (b) F (c) T (d) T

35. (a) T (b) F (c) F (d) F (e) F

    Large difference in acoustic impedance leads to more nerve clarity. Best view is seen if needle is perpendicular to ultrasound beam to minimise refraction and maximise reflection. This is the reason out of plane approach is preferred for deep-seated nerves.

36. (a) T (b) T (c) F (d) T (e) T

    Time gain compensation is the ability of operator to control gain independently at specified depth intervals.

37. (a) T   (b) T   (c) F   (d) T   (e) T

    Axial resolution is seen when two structures lie parallel
    to the ultrasound beam. High-frequency transducer
    probes offer high resolution at expense of low tissue
    penetration.

38. (a) T   (b) T   (c) T   (d) F   (e) T

39. (a) T   (b) T   (c) F   (d) T

    Tendons are more ordered than nerves, and anisotropic
    effects are seen with angle changes as small as 2°.

40. (a) T   (b) T   (c) T   (d) T   (e) F

    Spatial compound imaging is the steering of beam in
    different directions to help visualise needle tip. Needle
    visualisation is better with deeper blocks as back scatter
    from needle is received by transducer rather than a
    strong specular reflection.

41. (a) T   (b) T   (c) F   (d) F   (e) T

    Lateral resolution is improved by adjusting focus.
    Ultrasound beam first converges to a point called as
    Fresnel zone and then diverges (Fraunhofer zone).

42. (a) T   (b) F   (c) T   (d) T   (e) T

    Both undergain and overgain can contribute to artefact.
    When a structure has a larger attenuation coefficient
    than the tissue that lies deep to it, deeper tissue appears
    less echogenic than normal, e.g. under ribs, under
    vertebral spines.

43. (a) T   (b) F   (c) T   (d) T   (e) F

    Reverberation artefact is seen when needle is
    perpendicular and incidence decreases if angle
    decreases less than 90°. Multiple reverberation
    artefacts can cause image disturbance leading to

comet-tail sign. Ultrasound waves oscillate back and forth within the lumen of the needle shaft, and needle appears deep because time has elapsed for ultrasound waves to return to the probe. Decreasing gain can darken duplicate image and decrease reverberation artefact.

44. (a) T   (b) T   (c) F   (d) T   (e) F

Increase in amperage leads to increase sensitivity. This is useful in cutaneous electrodes for monitoring neuromuscular function.

45. (a) T   (b) F   (c) T   (d) T   (e) T

Short pulse impulses are used for nerve localisation (0.05–1 ms).

46. (a) T   (b) T   (c) F   (d) T   (e) T

Conduction gel is not required, but conduction is enhanced by cleaning and removing oil. Indentation decreases the distance between nerve and probe and decreases resistance.

47. (a) T   (b) T   (c) T   (d) F   (e) F

Both lower and upper limb injections are benefitted. Multiple injections decrease latency of blocks and decrease time of onset.

48. (a) T   (b) T   (c) F   (d) T   (e) T

In children, mostly hockey stick probes with surface length of 25 mm are used. Children are more at risk of local anaesthetic toxicity because deficient $\alpha 1$ acid glycoprotein and albumin.

49. (a) F   (b) F   (c) F   (d) T   (e) T

Physical examination alone is imprecise in localisation of levels in 70–80 % of patients. Ligamentum flavum and dura mater appear hyperechoic. Epidural space and cerebrospinal fluid are hypoechoic.

50. (a) F   (b) F   (c) F   (d) F   (e) T

The electrically conducting connection extends to tip only. 17- to 20-G needle is required for inserting catheters. Local anaesthetic or saline is injected in non-stimulating technique and is not required with stimulating catheters. Catheter is tunnelled and a skin bridge is made for easy removal for short-term use. For prolonged infusions (>7 days), tunnelling without skin bridge is done to avoid infection.

3 Pharmacology

1. Nerve cells:
   (a) Motor cells can arise from either somatic or autonomic system.
   (b) Alpha motor neurons innervate intrafusal fibres.
   (c) Sensory neurons are either somatic or visceral.
   (d) Both myelinated and unmyelinated fibres occur in PNS.
   (e) A myelinated fibre is surrounded by lemmocyte.

2. Peripheral nerves:
   (a) Epineurium surrounds the outside of each peripheral nerve.
   (b) Endoneurium surrounds each fascicle.
   (c) Tactile fibres are medium sized and myelinated.
   (d) Pain fibres are more heavy than tactile fibres.
   (e) All olfactory nerve filaments are unmyelinated.

3. Axons:
   (a) Large axons are myelinated.
   (b) Axons involved with proprioception are largest in sensory axons.
   (c) Unmyelinated c fibres forms autonomic fibres.
   (d) Type A fibres are myelinated fibres of spinal nerves.
   (e) C fibres conduct impulses at 2 m/s.

4. Axon:
   (a) Is the largest process of a nerve body.
   (b) Schwann cells can generate electrical stimulus.
   (c) Axon is only surrounded by Schwann cells.

R. Gupta, D. Patel, *Multiple Choice Questions in Regional Anaesthesia*,
DOI 10.1007/978-3-642-31257-1_3, © Springer-Verlag Berlin Heidelberg 2013

(d) Axoplasm contains cisternae of smooth endoplasmic reticulum.

(e) Nerve fibres always branch at nodes of Ranvier.

5. Schwann cells:
   (a) Axon regeneration is dependent on Schwann cells.
   (b) Main function is to provide nutrition and maintain ionic state.
   (c) Are derived from neural crest.
   (d) Grow by mitotic division.
   (e) Lack basal lamina.

6. Myelinated axons:
   (a) Axons <0.2 μ do not stimulate myelin formation.
   (b) There is a space in continuity with extracellular space at node of Ranvier where there is no myelin.
   (c) Myelin incisura are seen on longitudinal sections of myelinated nerve fibres.
   (d) Lipofuscin is normally seen in Schwann cells.
   (e) Schwann cells contain collagen types III, IV and V.

7. Unmyelinated axons:
   (a) Are usually <1.0 μ in diameter.
   (b) There are no nodes of Ranvier.
   (c) They are usually between 200 and 500 μm in length.
   (d) Pi granules are seen.
   (e) Myelin-associated glycoprotein is absent.

8. Connective tissue sheath of peripheral nerves:
   (a) Epineurium is present all around nerve fibres.
   (b) Perineurium consists of concentric layers of flattened cells separated by a layer of collagen.
   (c) Endoneurium may form two layers.
   (d) The predominant cell in endoneurium is a fibroblast.
   (e) Epineurium and endoneurium lack basal lamina.

9. Local anaesthetics:
   (a) Contain aromatic ring and an amine at the end of the molecule.
   (b) A hydrocarbon chain separates them.
   (c) There is always an amide link.
   (d) Cocaine is the only naturally occurring ester local anaesthetic.
   (e) Ropivacaine is the only single enantiomer local anaesthetic.

10. Voltage-gated sodium channels:
   (a) Contains two larger α subunits and one or two smaller β subunits.
   (b) External surface of α subunit is heavily glycosylated.
   (c) Congenital long QT syndrome is due to mutation in sodium channel.
   (d) All sodium channel alpha subunits will bind local anaesthetics similarly.
   (e) B subunits are the site of ion conduction and local anaesthetic binding.

11. Blocking of impulses in a nerve fibre:
   (a) Both conduction and local anaesthetic inhibition of conduction is same in myelinated and nonmyelinated fibres.
   (b) To block impulses in myelinated fibres, it is necessary to block at least three nodes of Ranvier.
   (c) Nonmyelinated fibres are relatively resistant to local anaesthetic.
   (d) Multiple sclerosis is due to alteration in sodium channels.
   (e) The concentration of local anaesthetic required to produce nerve block decreases as the length of nerve exposed to local anaesthetic increase.

12. Mechanism of action of local anaesthetics:
    (a) Skeletal muscle nerve fibres forms gate quicker than cardiac fibres.
    (b) Repetitive depolarisation may increase the affinity of sodium channels to local anaesthetics.
    (c) Only local anaesthetics inhibits sodium channels.
    (d) Potency of local anaesthetic increases with increased molecular weight and increased lipid solubility.
    (e) Speed of onset of local anaesthetics depends on pKa.

13. All are true except:
    (a) Local anaesthetics block smaller diameter fibres at lower concentration as compared to larger fibres of the same type.
    (b) Unmyelinated fibres are easily blocked as compared to the myelinated fibres.
    (c) Ropivacaine is selective for sensory fibres.
    (d) Onset of anaesthesia is fastest when injected subcutaneously as compared to plexus block.
    (e) Epinephrine increases local anaesthetic duration by increasing the duration of intraneural concentration of local anaesthetics.

14. All are true about local anaesthetics except:
    (a) Local anaesthetics have greater potency at basic pH.
    (b) Addition of sodium bicarbonate to local anaesthetics has no effect.
    (c) Sensitivity to local anaesthetics decreases in pregnancy.
    (d) Albumin is the primary local anaesthetic-binding protein.
    (e) Patients with right to left shunting are resistant to toxic effects of local anaesthetic.

15. Local anaesthetic metabolism:
    (a) Pseudocholinesterase causes hydrolysis of esters in blood.
    (b) Amides are metabolised by kidneys.
    (c) Glycine xylidide and monoethylglycinexylidide are metabolites of lidocaine.
    (d) Prilocaine causes methemoglobinemia.
    (e) B agonists and H2 antagonists can decrease amide clearance.

16. Side effects of local anaesthetic:
    (a) Local anaesthetic toxicity may increase excitation of CNS followed by depression.
    (b) Local anaesthetics produce dose-dependent myocardial depression.
    (c) Allergic reactions are more common with ester type local anaesthetics.
    (d) Cauda equina syndrome has been attributed to metabisulfite.
    (e) Lidocaine 5% permanently interrupts conduction when applied to isolated nerves.

17. Local anaesthetic toxicity:
    (a) Epileptics have increased susceptibility to local anaesthetic toxicity.
    (b) Primary site of cardiovascular toxicity is endocardium.
    (c) Methemoglobinemia is due to ferrous iron formation.
    (d) Tissue toxicity may be seen.
    (e) Infants are more resistant to local anaesthetic toxicity.

18. Treatment of local anaesthetic toxicity (intralipid):
    (a) It is 20 % fat emulsion.
    (b) It is acidic.
    (c) Has a high calorific value.

(d) Has higher osmolality.

(e) Mean particle size in emulsion is 0.5 μm.

19. Intralipid:

  (a) Bolus dose is 1.5 ml/kg.

  (b) Infusion should be started at the rate of 2.5 ml/kg/min.

  (c) Effective chest compressions help in better therapeutic effect.

  (d) Decrease in blood pressure is an indication to stop infusion.

  (e) Maximum dose of 8 ml/kg is recommended.

20. Chirality:

  (a) Local anaesthetics can exist as mirror images of each other.

  (b) Isomers of same compound will have same biological activities.

  (c) Depends on the direction that a molecule rotates polarised light.

  (d) Most anaesthetic drugs are racemic mixtures.

  (e) Both ropivacaine and S bupivacaine are chiral.

21. Physiochemical properties of local anaesthetics:

  (a) Ropivacaine is structurally related to mepivacaine and bupivacaine.

  (b) Bupivacaine has a propyl group.

  (c) pK of ropivacaine is similar to bupivacaine.

  (d) Bupivacaine has greater motor blocking effects than ropivacaine.

  (e) Ropivacaine has short elimination half-life.

22. Ropivacaine:

  (a) Is a S enantiomer.

  (b) Has lower toxicity than bupivacaine.

  (c) Causes lesser motor blockade.

  (d) Can cause both cardio- and neurotoxicity.

  (e) Can cause vasoconstriction.

23. Levobupivacaine
    (a) Is less protein bound than bupivacaine.
    (b) Has lower volume of distribution than bupivacaine.
    (c) Has similar protein binding and lipid solubility to that of racemic bupivacaine.
    (d) Both L-bupivacaine and bupivacaine have equal elimination half-life.
    (e) L-bupivacaine is more toxic than bupivacaine.

24. Liposomal local anaesthetic delivery:
    (a) Is ideal as a career vehicle.
    (b) Lipophilic drugs can be attached to it.
    (c) The drug to phospholipid ratio is important in drug delivery.
    (d) Structure of liposomes can be strengthened.
    (e) Liposomal encapsulation of bupivacaine appears to offer protection against CNS and CVS side effects.

25. Neuraxial adjuvants:
    (a) Maximum incidence of pruritus is seen with sufentanil if given intrathecally.
    (b) Epinephrine given epidurally intensifies the block of bupivacaine along with increasing the duration of action.
    (c) Phenylephrine can cause transient neurological symptoms if given intrathecally.
    (d) Clonidine may cause more hypotension if given in upper thoracic epidural space.
    (e) Sodium bicarbonate is more effective on speed of onset with lidocaine and mepivacaine than bupivacaine or ropivacaine.

26. Opioids as adjuvants:
    (a) Exert action by modulating Aδ and c fibres.
    (b) Have no effect on sympathetic outflow.

     (c) Epidural fentanyl can decrease requirements for volatiles and intravenous fentanyl.

     (d) Opioids have minimal effect on dorsal root axons.

     (e) Fentanyl has similar mechanism of action when given as a bolus epidurally or as an infusion.

27. Vasopressors as adjuvants:
    (a) Phenylephrine is used as 1 % solution.
    (b) Epinephrine extends the effect of block by 100 %.
    (c) Slow vascular resorption is seen with vasopressors.
    (d) Association with spinal cord ischaemia is seen.
    (e) Systemic toxicity is reduced.

28. Epinephrine
    (a) Can reduce peak blood levels.
    (b) Provide more reliable block.
    (c) Intensifies analgesia and anaesthesia.
    (d) Is used solely due to its vasoconstricting effect.
    (e) At low doses stimulates both $\alpha 1$ and $\alpha 2$ receptors.

29. Adrenaline for epidural analgesia:
    (a) Typical concentration used is 1:250,000.
    (b) Commercially available mixtures are alkaline to preserve potency.
    (c) All anaesthetic agents react favourably with the addition of adrenaline.
    (d) Effect of epinephrine is due to constriction of epidural venous plexus and decreased blood flow and slower uptake of local anaesthetic.
    (e) Adrenaline addition can prolong discharge times and delay bladder function.

30. Alpha2 adrenergic agonists:
    (a) Clonidine exerts effect by blocking sodium channels.
    (b) Binds to substantia gelatinosa and brainstem nuclei.

(c) Increases acetylcholine and noradrenaline in CSF.
(d) Are hydrophilic.
(e) Yohimbine reverses analgesic effects of clonidine.

31. Clonidine administered neuraxially:
    (a) Directly inhibits preganglionic sympathetic neurons in spinal cord.
    (b) Drop in blood pressure is dependent on whether injected in mid-thoracic or upper thoracic region.
    (c) Can decrease chronotropic drive.
    (d) At higher concentration, can cause vasoconstriction.
    (e) Can produce segmental hypoalgesia when administered in epidural space.

32. Alkalinisation of local anaesthetics:
    (a) Increases the difference between pH and pKa, thus increasing the speed of onset.
    (b) Ropivacaine does not show faster onset with alkalinisation.
    (c) Solutions containing epinephrine respond best to alkalinisation.
    (d) Carbonate salts of local anaesthetic are shown to have more rapid onset of epidural blockade than standard chloride preparations.
    (e) Carbonated drugs induce more hypotension.

33. Neostigmine given intrathecally:
    (a) Inhibits breakdown of acetylcholine in spinal cord.
    (b) Has a high incidence of nausea and vomiting.
    (c) Can cause increased heart rate and respiratory rate.
    (d) Can cause side effects like incontinence and motor weakness.
    (e) Enhances motor and sensory blockade if added to bupivacaine.

34. Ketamine:
    (a) Is a non-competitive antagonist of NMDA receptors.
    (b) Is available as a racemic mixture.
    (c) Can be used as both intrathecally and epidurally.
    (d) Uses include pre-emptive analgesia and treatment of chronic neuropathic pain.
    (e) Psychomimetic side effects are not seen if injected with bupivacaine.

35. Nerve roots:
    (a) α Fibres are purely motor.
    (b) β fibres are preganglionic.
    (c) As a rule, large myelinated fibres require large amount of local anaesthetic to block conduction.
    (d) β fibres are first to be blocked and last to recover.
    (e) The onset time is influenced by molecule's pKa and diffusibility.

36. Local anaesthetic solutions:
    (a) The ability to cross cell membrane depends on molecular weight and lipid solubility of molecule.
    (b) All local anaesthetics have almost same molecular weight.
    (c) pKa can be modified by warming or adding sodium bicarbonate
    (d) Local tissue acidosis can increase the speed of onset.
    (e) Minimum effective concentration relates to potency.

37. Cm of a local anaesthetic:
    (a) Is related to potency.
    (b) Is constant for all sizes of nerve fibre.
    (c) Smaller nerve fibres with slower conduction are more sensitive to blockade.

(d) Three consecutive nodes of Ranvier need to be blocked to produce a complete nerve block.

(e) Differential sensory-motor blockade is seen more with lipophilic agents.

38. Local anaesthetic blockade:
   (a) The fastest onset of action is seen with mepivacaine.
   (b) Maximum dose of mepivacaine is 600 mg
   (c) The concentration of ropivacaine used is 0.07–0.1 %.
   (d) Duration of action of L-bupivacaine is 4–8 h.
   (e) 0.2 % ropivacaine can be used for continuous analgesia.

39. Midazolam:
   (a) Forms most common group for conscious sedation.
   (b) Etomidate is particularly helpful in elderly patients.
   (c) Propofol is better option than midazolam and methohexital for adequate sedation.
   (d) A combination of midazolam and propofol provides a better combination with desired results.
   (e) Efficacy of remifentanil infusion is same as alfentanil infusion.

40. Supplementation of local anaesthetic:
   (a) Both propofol and midazolam can be used as self-administered agents.
   (b) Sevoflurane is required in high doses to supplement local anaesthetic.
   (c) Monitored anaesthesia care during sedation has been shown to be more effective for regional anaesthesia.
   (d) Paracoxib is the most effective analgesic of all COX inhibitors.

41. Local anaesthetics pharmacokinetics:
   (a) Distribution after injection is affected by baricity of drug.
   (b) Nonmyelinated nerve roots are immune to damage.

    (c) Blood flow will decrease the concentration of local anaesthetics.

    (d) Drugs may alter blood flow to spinal cord.

    (e) Elimination of local anaesthetics is by vascular absorption.

42. Local anaesthetic distribution:

    (a) Lidocaine is the most hyperbaric local anaesthetic.

    (b) Baricity depends upon the molecular structure.

    (c) Isobaric solutions have same density as cerebrospinal fluid.

    (d) Dose and volume are equally important in spread of local anaesthetic.

    (e) Hypobaric solution is useful in prone position surgery.

Answers

1. (a) T   (b) F   (c) T   (d) T   (e) T
   Alpha motor neurons innervate extrafusal fibres.
   Lemmocytes are also known as plasma membrane or
   Schwann cells.

2. (a) T   (b) F   (c) T   (d) F   (e) T
   Each fascicle is surrounded by perineurium.

3. (a) T   (b) T   (c) F   (d) T   (e) F

4. (a) T   (b) T   (c) F   (d) T   (e) T
   Axons propagate action potential. Schwann cells can
   generate long-lasting depolarising potential which slowly
   propagates. Axon cytoplasm is known as axoplasm.

5. (a) T   (b) T   (c) T   (d) T   (e) T

6. (a) F   (b) T   (c) T   (d) F   (e) T
   Axons <1.0 μ do not stimulate myelin formation. The
   space is known as periaxonal space of Klebs; myelin
   incisura are also known as Schmidt-Lanterman clefts. The
   larger the diameter of axon, the more are the clefts in
   Schwann cells. Lipofuscin increases with age.

7. (a) T   (b) T   (c) T   (d) F   (e) T
   Pi granules of Reich are seen in paranuclear cytoplasm in
   myelinated axons. Myelin-associated glycoprotein is
   responsible for myelination of axons and is absent in
   unmyelinated axons.

8. (a) F   (b) T   (c) T   (d) T   (e) T

Epineurium is the outermost sheath and is lacking around monofascicular nerves. Endoneurium has two layers. Outer layer is extraneural sheath of Key and Retzius which produces longitudinal fibres which are closely packed. Inner layer of Plenk and Laidlaw consists of fine collagen fibres which are randomly oriented.

9. (a) T   (b) T   (c) F   (d) T   (e) F

Ropivacaine and levobupivacaine are both S enantiomers.

10. (a) F   (b) T   (c) T   (d) T   (e) T

Sodium channel contains one larger and one or two smaller β units. Glycosylation orients the channel properly within the plasma membrane.

11. (a) F   (b) T   (c) T   (d) T   (e) T

Unmyelinated fibres are resistant to local anaesthetics due to dispersal of sodium channels throughout their plasma membrane. In multiple sclerosis, there is loss of clustering of sodium channels in axons.

12. (a) T   (b) T   (c) F   (d) T   (e) T

Gating is a process by which channels change from conducting to non-conducting fibres. It is seen due to movement of diploes in response to changes in potential. Use dependence is increased local anaesthetic inhibition of sodium currents with repetitive depolarisation. Apart from local anaesthetic, α2 agonists and tricyclic antidepressants also block sodium channels. Larger more lipophilic local anaesthetics permeate nerve membranes more readily and bind sodium channels with affinity. Uncharged ions have higher speed of onset.

13. (a) T   (b) F   (c) T   (d) T   (e) T

Bupivacaine also produces more rapid onset of sensory than motor block.

14. (a) T (b) F (c) F (d) F (e) F

    Increased fraction of local anaesthetic molecules is
    uncharged. Addition of sodium bicarbonate hastens
    onset of block. Sensitivity to local anaesthetics is
    increased in pregnancy. The spread of local anaesthetics
    is also increased in pregnancy. Main binding protein is
    α1 acid glycoprotein.

15. Amides are metabolised by liver. Lidocaine undergoes
    oxidative N-dealkylation by cytochrome CYP1A2 and
    CYP3A4. Prilocaine is metabolised to O-toluidine which
    causes methemoglobinemia. Amide clearance depends
    on hepatic blood, hepatic extraction and enzyme
    function. B agonists and H2 antagonists decrease hepatic
    blood flow.

16. Excitation is seen with seizures arising from amygdala.
    Myocardial depression is seen because of interference
    with calcium signalling within cardiac muscle.
    Lidocaine 5 % when applied to nerves permanently
    interrupts conduction because of increase in intracellu-
    lar calcium.

17. (a) F (b) F (c) F (d) T (e) T

    Local anaesthetic has anticonvulsant action and has
    been used for treatment of generalised tonic-clonic
    seizures. Primary site of local anaesthetic toxicity is
    myocardium. Methemoglobinemia is seen when ferrous
    iron in haemoglobin is oxidised to ferric form. Muscles
    and nerves are mainly affected.

18. (a) T (b) F (c) T (d) T (e) T

    It is made up of 20 % soya bean oil, 1.2 % egg yolk,
    phospholipids, 1.7 % glycerine and water for injection.
    Sodium hydroxide has been added to adjust the final pH
    to 8.0. Total calorific value is 3.0 kcal/ml of intralipid
    30 %. The osmolality is 310 mOsm/kg water.

19. (a) T (b) F (c) T (d) F (e) T

The bolus dose is 1.5 ml/kg over one minute. Infusion should be started at 0.25 ml/kg/min. Effective chest compressions are required for lipid circulation. The infusion should be increased to 0.5 ml/kg/min if blood pressure decreased.

20. (a) T (b) F (c) T (d) T (e) T

21. (a) T (b) F (c) T (d) T (e) T

Bupivacaine has butyl group, whereas ropivacaine has propyl group. The pH of ropivacaine is 8.07, and bupivacaine is 8.1. Bupivacaine is more lipid soluble which enhances its penetration into heavily myelinated, large motor neurons. Ropivacaine has short elimination half-life because of fast clearance.

22. (a) T (b) T (c) T (d) T (e) T

It is S enantiomer of 1-propyl-2',6' pipecoloxylidide. It is less toxic because of slower uptake. The drug is similar in efficacy to bupivacaine for pain relief but causes lesser motor blockade. This is because of high pKa (8.2) and low solubility. The drug preferentially blocks nerve fibres responsible for pain transmission (Aβ and C fibres) rather than the motor function. It can cause both neuro- and cardiotoxicity, though the incidence of cardiotoxicity is considerably reduced. It has a biphasic vascular effect, causing vasoconstriction at low concentration.

23. (a) F (b) T (c) T (d) F (e) F

L-bupivacaine has shorter half-life than bupivacaine.

24. (a) T (b) F (c) T (d) T (e) T

Liposomes are biocompatible, biodegradable and non-immunogenic. Both lipophilic and hydrophilic drugs can be attached to liposomes. A higher drug to phospholipid ratio allows more of the drug to be delivered with less lysosome, whereas a low drug to phospholipid ratio requires administration of a very large lipid load to achieve the desired drug effect. This may make it unsuitable to be used via subcutaneous route.

25. (a) F (b) F (c) T (d) T (e) T

The incidence of pruritus is maximum with fentanyl especially when given with procaine and 2-chlorprocaine. Epinephrine has no effect on the duration of action.

26. (a) T (b) F (c) F (d) T (e) F

Opioids have no effect on motor or sympathetic blockade but may reduce sympathetic flow via opioid receptors in the sympathetic ganglia, thereby eliciting hypotension. Epidural fentanyl can decrease requirements for volatile anaesthetics more than intravenous fentanyl. Fentanyl given as an epidural bolus produces segmental analgesia consistent with spinal levels of action. If given as an infusion, analgesia is mediated through systemic uptake and supraspinal effect. Similar effect is seen with alfentanil and sufentanil.

27. (a) T (b) F (c) T (d) T (e) T

Phenylephrine is used in 1 % solution. It extends the duration of effect of local anaesthetic by 30–100 %. Epinephrine extends the block by 40–50 %.

28. (a) T (b) T (c) T (d) F (e) F

Epinephrine also has effect on presynaptic adrenergic receptors that directly contributes to analgesia.

29. (a) F (b) F (c) F (d) T (e) T

Commercial adrenaline is used in concentration of 1:200,000 or 5 μg/ml. Mixtures are made acidic to preserve potency. This slows onset of blockade and inhibits vasoconstrictive actions of adrenaline. Ropivacaine has vasoconstrictive action and therefore intensifies block without prolonging the duration.

30. (a) F   (b) T   (c) T   (d) F   (e) T

Clonidine produces conduction blockade by attenuating Aδ and c fibre nociception thus increasing K conductance. Clonidine is α2 agonist and yohimbine is α2 antagonist.

31. (a) T   (b) T   (c) T   (d) T   (e) T

Upper thoracic dermatomes supply the heart and sympathetic preganglionic neurons and thus cause more hypotension. Clonidine activates presynaptic α2 receptors and inhibits release of noradrenaline from terminals of sympathetic nerves causing decreased chronotropic drive.

32. (a) F   (b) T   (c) T   (d) T   (e) T

Alkalinisation raises pH closer to pKa making more non-ionised molecule present thus increasing speed of onset. Epinephrine has pH dependant vasoconstricting actions.

33. (a) T   (b) T   (c) T   (d) T   (e) T

Acetylcholine causes spinal analgesia through stimulation of cholinergic receptors in substantia gelatinosa and superficial laminae of the dorsal horn of spinal cord.

34. (a) T   (b) T   (c) T   (d) T   (e) F

Ketamine is a non-competitive antagonist of NMDA receptors, but it also has actions at monoaminergic receptors, opioid receptors, voltage-sensitive calcium channels and muscarinic receptors. The S enantiomer is more potent at NMDA receptor. Ketamine can be used

both intrathecally and via epidural route, but there is a
high failure rate when used intrathecally.

35. (a) F   (b) T   (c) T   (d) T   (e) T

A Fibres are further divided into Aα, Aβ and Aγ which
are all myelinated. Aδ fibres are sensory which respond
to pressure and distension. Large fibres require large
amount of local anaesthetic to block conduction as a
rule except β fibres of autonomic system which even
though myelinated require minimum concentration to
block them. This is the reason why sympathetic block is
observed before the block of other fibres.

36. (a) T   (b) T   (c) T   (d) F   (e) T

Warming or adding bicarbonate can increase unionised
solution. Local tissue acidosis can cause acidosis, thus
increasing ionised form and delaying the speed of onset.
Cm-minimum anaesthetic concentration reduces the
action potential of a nerve fibre bathed in a solution with
a 7.2–7.4 pH and stimulated with a 30 Hz current by
50 % within 5 min.

37. (a) T   (b) F   (c) T   (d) T   (e) T

Lower concentration of local anaesthetic blocks small
fibres and causes differential sensory-motor blockade.

38. (a) T   (b) T   (c) F   (d) T   (e) T

Both lignocaine and mepivacaine have fast onset of
action. The concentration of ropivacaine used is 0.75–1 %.

39. (a) T   (b) T   (c) T   (d) T   (e) F

Etomidate can be given as a continuous infusion and has
minimal cardiovascular side effects. Propofol is
equivalent in effect to midazolam and methohexital but
with less incidence of sedation, amnesia and nausea and
vomiting.

40. (a) T   (b) F   (c) T   (d) F

41. (a) T   (b) F   (c) T   (d) T   (e) F

    Nonmyelinated nerve roots are more likely to be damaged by local anaesthetics. The more is the blood flow, the faster is the clearance of the local anaesthetic. Local anaesthetics affect spinal cord blood flow. Tetracaine increases blood flow whereas it is decreased by lidocaine and bupivacaine.

42. (a) T   (b) F   (c) T   (d) F   (e) T

    Baricity is achieved by adding glucose or dextrose to local anaesthetic. Bupivacaine has a density of 1.0207, while density of lidocaine is 1.0265. The density of CSF is 1.000, and the density of water is 0.9930. The dosage of local anaesthetics affects spread of local anaesthetics more than the volume.

4 The Upper Extremity

1. Cervical plexus:
   (a) Formed by anterior divisions of four upper cervical nerves.
   (b) Easy to locate as it lies superficial to sternocleidomastoid muscle.
   (c) All four nerves send branches to accessory nerve.
   (d) C3 supplies tragus of ear.
   (e) Upper part of ear is supplied by minor occipital nerve.

2. Deep cervical plexus block:
   (a) Sternocleidomastoid anterior border is one of the landmarks.
   (b) A line connecting the mastoid process and C6 tubercle is required.
   (c) Even one injection at level of C3 on the above line is enough.
   (d) 3–5 ml of local anaesthetic is required per level.
   (e) Ropivacaine has been shown to be the most effective for carotid endarterectomy.

3. Deep cervical block:
   (a) Needle should be inserted with a caudal orientation.
   (b) Transverse process is contacted at 3–4 cm in most patients.
   (c) Complications include cervical cord injury, carotid and vertebral artery puncture.

R. Gupta, D. Patel, *Multiple Choice Questions in Regional Anaesthesia*,
DOI 10.1007/978-3-642-31257-1_4, © Springer-Verlag Berlin Heidelberg 2013

(d) Cervical nerves are just anterior to transverse process.

(e) Carotid surgery can be done under cervical plexus block.

4. Blockade of superficial cervical plexus:
   (a) Individual nerves emerge from posterior border of sternocleidomastoid.
   (b) Greater occipital nerve is a direct branch from C2.
   (c) Supraclavicular nerves are formed from C3 and C4.
   (d) Needle is inserted midpoint between mastoid process and transverse process of C6.
   (e) Transient ischaemic attacks and recurrent laryngeal nerve blocks are known complications.

5. Cervical paravertebral block:
   (a) The needle insertion point is at level of apex of the V formed by trapezius and levator scapulae muscles.
   (b) Angle of needle insertion is anterolateral and cranial.
   (c) Catheter can be inserted for continuous analgesia.
   (d) Is sufficient on its own for shoulder surgery.
   (e) Ideal for continuous catheter analgesia as catheters follow nerve roots.

6. Complications of cervical paravertebral block:
   (a) Horner syndrome is seen in 40 % patients
   (b) Most common organism in infection of catheters is streptococcus.
   (c) Neck pain is a common complication.
   (d) Subclavian artery puncture is not possible.
   (e) Contralateral epidural spread can be seen.

7. Brachial plexus:
   (a) Formed by ventral rami of C5–T1.
   (b) Supplies all the motor and sensory function of shoulder.

(c) Supplies shoulder joint.
(d) Rhomboids and levator scapulae are not supplied by brachial plexus.
(e) Serratus anterior is supplied by C567.

8. Brachial plexus blockade:
   (a) Interscalene block is at the level of the roots.
   (b) Lower trunk is incompletely blocked with interscalene approach.
   (c) Sensory block may be seen up to C2 with interscalene block.
   (d) Supraclavicular nerves preferentially blocks axillary nerve.
   (e) Multiple-injection technique at the level of axilla increases the chances of success by 90 %.

9. Brachial plexus blockade (classic Winnie's technique):
   (a) Interscalene groove is one of the landmarks.
   (b) Needle is inserted perpendicularly.
   (c) Original technique relied on hitting transverse process.
   (d) A paraesthesia to the shoulder is confirmation of adequate position of needle.
   (e) Cervical cord injection with paraplegia has been observed with wrong technique.

10. Brachial plexus block (posterior approach):
    (a) C6 and C7 forms the landmarks.
    (b) Point of needle insertion is 7 cm lateral to interspinous line.
    (c) Loss of resistance is felt as interscalene space is entered.
    (d) It is equivalent to paravertebral approach to brachial plexus.
    (e) Muscles traversed are trapezius, splenius cervicis and levator scapulae.

11. Brachial plexus block (Meier approach):
     (a) Decreases the risk of complication.
     (b) Same landmarks as Winnie's approach.
     (c) Needle is inserted perpendicular.
     (d) Catheter placement is easy.
     (e) Point of needle insertion is cranial to cricoid cartilage.

12. Brachial plexus block (Borgeat):
     (a) Interscalene groove is an important landmark.
     (b) Point of insertion is 5 mm above cricoid cartilage.
     (c) Needle is directed caudally.
     (d) Is good for single-shot nerve block.
     (e) Positioning of patient is the same as Winnie's block.

13. Brachial plexus block (Pippa's technique)
     (a) Is done in a sitting position.
     (b) The puncture point is midpoint of a line joining C5 and C6.
     (c) The target is ipsilateral to the cricoid cartilage.
     (d) Ipsilateral block of phrenic nerve is seen commonly.
     (e) Horner's syndrome can be seen.

14. Response to nerve stimulation in interscalene block:
     (a) Local twitch of neck muscles means needle is moving in the right plane.
     (b) Pectoralis muscle twitch is acceptable.
     (c) Twitch of scapula is seen as confirmatory of appropriate position.
     (d) Trapezius stimulation is seen with posterior placement of needle to brachial plexus.
     (e) Twitch of biceps and triceps is acceptable.

15. Continuous interscalene brachial plexus block:
     (a) Patient positioning is same as single-shot injection.
     (b) Needle is inserted perpendicularly.

   (c) Supraclavicular nerve can be blocked as rescue
       nerve.
   (d) For lower shoulder surgery, intercostobrachial nerve
       should be blocked.
   (e) Catheter should be placed 2–3 cm distal to the needle.

16. Side effects of interscalene block:
   (a) Most common side effect is ipsilateral
       hemidiaphragmatic paresis.
   (b) The incidence of hoarseness is 1 %.
   (c) Bezold-Jarisch reflex is rare.
   (d) Modified lateral approach has got the least
       complication rate.
   (e) Horner's syndrome consists of enophthalmos,
       proptosis and hyperaemia of conjunctiva.

17. Supraclavicular block:
   (a) Can be used for shoulder surgery.
   (b) Suprascapular nerve arises from the upper trunk
       just proximal to origin of anterior and posterior
       division of trunk.
   (c) Pleural dome is seen both lateral and medial to
       anterior scalene muscle.
   (d) C8T1 can be missed if injection is not done
       immediately in the vicinity.
   (e) Brachial plexus crosses clavicle at or near its
       midpoint.

18. Landmark technique for supraclavicular block:
   (a) The landmarks are lateral insertion of
       sternocleidomastoid muscle, clavicle and patient's
       midline.
   (b) Point of insertion is 2 cm above insertion of
       sternocleidomastoid.
   (c) Needle is inserted perpendicularly and then parallel
       to midline.

    (d) Twitches at 0.8 mA can be accepted for injections.
    (e) Needle should never be inserted more than 1 cm.

19. Complications of supraclavicular nerve block:
    (a) Phrenic nerve block is seen in 100 % of patients.
    (b) Pneumothorax is rare.
    (c) Pneumothorax can be a delayed complication.
    (d) Neurologic injuries are rare.
    (e) Phrenic nerve block is associated with respiratory dysfunction.

20. Infraclavicular block:
    (a) Can be used for entire arm surgery.
    (b) Special positioning of patient is required.
    (c) Coagulopathy is a relative contraindication.
    (d) Block is at the level of roots.
    (e) Cords surround subclavian artery below clavicle.

21. Brachial plexus block below clavicle:
    (a) The block is at level of cords.
    (b) Cords surround axillary artery.
    (c) Lateral cord is superior, medial cord in between and posterior cord the deepest.
    (d) Radial nerve is formed by both medial and lateral cord
    (e) Musculocutaneous nerve is close to the lateral cord.

22. Brachial plexus:
    (a) Lateral cord is formed by anterior divisions of C567.
    (b) Anterior division of lower trunk forms posterior cord.
    (c) Axillary is a terminal branch of brachial plexus.
    (d) Thoracodorsal nerve supplies latissimus dorsi.
    (e) Axillary nerve is a pure sensory nerve.

23. Brachial plexus (lateral cord):
    (a) Provides motor innervations to flexor muscles of arm.
    (b) Has no innervations to the thumb
    (c) On stimulation, response is shown as extension of fingers.
    (d) Musculocutaneous nerve is purely motor below the elbow.
    (e) Stimulation of musculocutaneous nerve is a reliable indicator of lateral cord.

24. Brachial plexus (posterior cord):
    (a) Involved in upper arm movement and shoulder movement.
    (b) Distal stimulation causes abduction of thumb and extension of wrist and fingers.
    (c) Lies superficial to lateral cord in relation to axillary artery.
    (d) Elbow flexion with radial deviation of wrists represents stimulation of brachioradialis muscle and can be accepted for injection.
    (e) Brachioradialis is innervated by radial nerve.

25. Brachial cord (medical cord):
    (a) Innervates skin of medial surface of forearm.
    (b) Ulnar nerve supplies lateral two interossei.
    (c) Ulnar nerve is responsible for thumb opposition.
    (d) Ulnar nerve does not provide sensory innervation to hand.
    (e) Wrist flexion is reliable indicator of median nerve.

26. Infraclavicular block (modified raj approach):
    (a) Landmark is a line from jugular fossa to clavicular acromial joint
    (b) The insertion point is 5 cm inferior to midpoint of above line.

(c) Angle of needle is 45–60° towards point of palpation of axillary artery.

(d) Can be done with patient sitting up.

(e) Has high success rate.

27. Vertical infraclavicular block:
    (a) Landmarks are midpoint of a line from middle of fossa jugularis and ventral process of acromion.
    (b) Needle is inserted 5 cm below the clavicle.
    (c) Keep the needle medially to avoid pneumothorax.
    (d) A more lateral puncture is more successful.
    (e) 100-mm needle should be used.

28. Coracoid approach (infraclavicular block):
    (a) Needle is inserted 2 cm inferior and medial to coracoids process.
    (b) Needle is inserted at an angle of 45°.
    (c) Endpoint is needle hitting the tip of coracoid process.
    (d) Plexus is normally encountered at 3–4 cm.

29. Axillary plexus is popular because:
    (a) Low risk of serious complications.
    (b) Of superior location.
    (c) Of good analgesia of upper arm.
    (d) Of suitability for tourniquet.
    (e) Of ease of procedure.

30. Axillary plexus block:
    (a) Can be used for surgery of wrist, forearm and hands.
    (b) Axillary lymphadenopathy is a relative contraindication.
    (c) Best avoided in neurological diseases.
    (d) Can be used for shoulder surgery.
    (e) Tourniquet use is contraindicated.

31. Axillary brachial plexus block:
    (a) All terminal nerves of brachial plexus accompany artery in axilla.
    (b) Musculocutaneous and median nerves lie superior to artery and ulnar and radial nerve lie inferior to the artery.
    (c) Midhumeral approach can be used for both ulnar and radial nerves.
    (d) Median nerve is more superficial than musculocutaneous nerve.
    (e) Radial and musculocutaneous nerves are found behind the artery.

32. Axillary brachial plexus block:
    (a) Coracobrachialis forms one of the landmarks.
    (b) Arm should be abducted to 90°.
    (c) Single injection axillary block is fastest and most reliable.
    (d) Elbow flexion can be accepted for injection.
    (e) Extension of wrist and hand indicates that needle is below the artery.

33. Axillary plexus block:
    (a) Both medium and ulnar nerves can result in wrist and finger flexion.
    (b) Median nerve will result in forearm supination.
    (c) Double-injection technique includes injection above and below the artery.
    (d) Multiple-injection technique gives the best results.
    (e) Transraterial is the most commonly used technique.

34. Axillary block (midhumeral approach):
    (a) Midhumeral approach is same as multi-injection axillary approach.
    (b) Midhumeral approach has a lower risk of neurological complications.
    (c) Can be used to supplement axillary block.

(d) Failure of midhumeral block can be supplemented with axillary block.

(e) Axillary block is better than infraclavicular approach in elbow block.

35. Complications of axillary block:
    (a) Toxicity due to absorption of local anaesthetics becomes symptomatic more than 1 h after surgery.
    (b) Symptoms of nerve damage appear within 1 h.
    (c) Most nerve injuries are neuropraxias.
    (d) Local anaesthetic should not be injected if motor stimulation is seen with current strength <0.2 mA.
    (e) High resistance is expected on injection within neurovascular sheath.

36. Ulnar nerve block at elbow:
    (a) Done in supine position.
    (b) Medial epicondyle is one of the landmarks.
    (c) Paraesthesia elicitation is required.
    (d) Ulnar nerve lies deep.
    (e) Medial half of fingers are blocked in hand.

37. Wrist block:
    (a) Radial nerve has no sensory innervations in hand.
    (b) Hypothenar muscles are supplied by median nerve.
    (c) Median nerve supplies skin of lateral three and half digits.
    (d) Ulnar nerve supplies all lumbricals.
    (e) Radial nerve is medial to radial artery.

38. Anatomical landmarks for wrist block:
    (a) Superficial branch of median nerve lies over anatomical snuff box.
    (b) Median nerve is between palmaris longus and flexor carpi radialis.
    (c) Ulnar nerve passes between ulnar artery and flexor carpi ulnaris.

(d) Radial nerve is a field block.
(e) Anatomical snuff box is formed by extensor pollicis brevis and extensor pollicis longus.

39. Radial nerve block at wrist:
    (a) Is essentially a field block.
    (b) Is a subcutaneous injection.
    (c) Single injection suffices for blocking radial nerve.
    (d) Dorsal sensory branches exits between brachioradialis and extensor carpi radialis longus.
    (e) Endpoint is when needle touches Lister's tubercle.

40. Ulnar nerve block at wrist:
    (a) Ulnar nerve lies lateral to flexor carpi ulnaris.
    (b) Nerve is approached medially just above styloid process.
    (c) Cutaneous branch of ulnar nerve is blocked above the tendon.
    (d) Dorsal sensory branch of ulnar nerve is blocked at the level of ulnar styloid.

41. Median nerve block at wrist:
    (a) Blocked by inserting needle between tendons of flexor carpi radialis and flexor carpi ulnaris.
    (b) A fascial click is indicative of appropriate position.
    (c) Twitches obtained characteristically show forearm pronation.
    (d) Epinephrine helps in usage of lower concentration in digital blocks.
    (e) Systemic toxicity is rare after wrist block.

42. Transthecal digital block:
    (a) Local anaesthetic injection is in flexor tendon sheaths.
    (b) Point of entry is distal palmar crease.
    (c) Needle should be inserted perpendicularly to skin surface.

(d) Good for anaesthesia of entire digit with one injection.

(e) Proximal pressure is applied to promote diffusion.

43. Supraclavicular nerve block;

(a) Supraclavicular nerve provides sensory innervations to the cape of the shoulder.

(b) Can be used solely for carotid artery surgery.

(c) The nerve is derived from ventral rami of C3 and C4.

(d) A single injection at anterior border of sternocleidomastoid is sufficient.

(e) Complications include internal jugular vein puncture.

44. Suprascapular nerve block:

(a) Good for arthroscopic and shoulder surgery.

(b) Arises from superior trunk of brachial plexus.

(c) The nerve provides major cutaneous innervations over posterior shoulder.

(d) Stimulation causes motor response of external shoulder rotation.

(e) Pneumothorax is a known complication.

45. Suprascapular nerve block:

(a) The nerve receives fibres from C5 and C6 nerve fibres.

(b) Supplies muscles but no joints.

(c) Patient should be supine with neutral head position.

(d) Acromion forms one of the landmarks.

(e) Transient weakness of muscles may be seen.

46. Intercostobrachial nerve block:

(a) Is used for surgery involving medial/posterior upper arm.

(b) Is good for blocking ischaemic compressive component of tourniquet pain.

   (c) Arises from T2 nerve root.
   (d) Nerve can be blocked by simply depositing a subcutaneous line of local anaesthetic superior and inferior along axillary crease.
   (e) Complications are rare.

47. Intravenous regional anaesthesia:
   (a) Can be performed for outpatient surgical procedures.
   (b) One intravenous drip can be used both for anaesthesia and emergency drugs.
   (c) The pressure in the cuff should be equal to the systolic pressure.
   (d) The injection should be done slowly.
   (e) After the procedure the deflation should be done intermittently.

48. Intravenous regional anaesthesia:
   (a) Local anaesthetic with vasoconstrictor actions should not be used.
   (b) Prilocaine has the least toxic profile to be used for this block.
   (c) Has fast onset of action.
   (d) Can be used for operations up to 4 hours long.
   (e) Does not provide a blood free operating area.

Answers

1. (a) T (b) F (c) F (d) F (e) T

Cervical plexus is formed by anterior divisions C1 to C4. The plexus lies deep to sternocleidomastoid muscle. Only third and fourth nerves send branches to accessory nerve. Tragus of ear is supplied by auriculotemporal nerve.

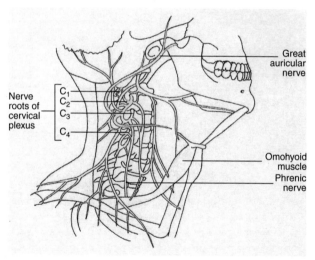

Cervical plexus

2. (a) F (b) T (c) T (d) T (e) T

The landmarks for deep cervical plexus block are posterior border of sternocleidomastoid, mastoid process and Chassaignac's tubercle.

3. (a) F (b) F (c) T (d) T (e) F

Needle should be inserted perpendicularly with a slight caudal angulation. The needle should never be inserted cephalad to avoid spinal cord. Transverse process is contacted at 1–2 cm. Cervical plexus lies anterior to transverse process. Carotid surgery can be done with cervical plexus block but also requires glossopharyngeal nerve block which is achieved by injecting into carotid sheath.

4. (a) T   (b) F   (c) T   (d) T   (e) T

Lesser occipital nerve is a direct branch of C2. Complications of superficial cervical plexus block are transient ischaemic attacks, recurrent laryngeal nerve blocks, infection, haematoma, phrenic nerve palsy, local anaesthetic toxicity and intrathecal injection.

5. (a) T   (b) F   (c) T   (d) F   (e) F

Angle of needle is anteromedial and 30° caudal and is aimed towards suprasternal notch or cricoid cartilage until C6 transverse process is encountered. Catheters curl up at the level of nerve roots, so should not be inserted >3–5 cm beyond the needle tip. Deeper insertion may cause knot formation.

6. (a) T   (b) F   (c) T   (d) F   (e) T

Up to 8 % of patients complain of dyspnoea in recovery. Most common organisms causing infection are Staphylococcus aureus and Staphylococcus epidermidis. Subclavian artery puncture is possible by posterior approach.

7. (a) T   (b) F   (c) T   (d) F   (e) T

Brachial plexus is formed by C5 to T1. Contribution from C4 makes it a prefixed plexus, while a contribution from T2 makes it a post-fixed plexus. It supplies all the motor and sensory functions of shoulder except cephalad portion of shoulder. Rhomboids and levator scapulae are supplied by dorsal scapular nerve (C4/5). Serratus anterior is supplied by long thoracic nerve.

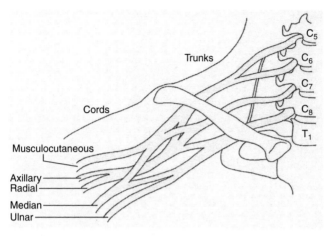

Brachial plexus

8. (a) T   (b) T   (c) T   (d) T   (e) T

Supraclavicular approach preferentially blocks axillary, radial and musculocutaneous nerve, whereas ulnar and median nerve blockade is incomplete.

9. (a) F   (b) T   (c) F   (d) F   (e) T

Landmarks are cricoids cartilage and sternocleidomastoid. Initial technique relied on paraesthesia. Paraesthesia elicited should always be below shoulder as if experienced in the shoulder could be because of stimulation of suprascapular nerve.

10. (a) T   (b) F   (c) T   (d) T   (e) T

Point of needle insertion is 3 cm lateral to interspinous line. Loss of resistance is seen after penetration through posterior and middle scalene muscles. The landmarks for posterior approach are (1) midpoint between cutaneous projections of spinal processes of sixth and seventh cervical vertebrae and (2) cutaneous projections of supero-exterior edge of trapezius muscle-aponeurotic line. Point of needle insertion is at the intersection of point 1 with point 2.

11. (a) T   (b) T   (c) F   (d) T   (e) T

The needle is inserted at an angle of 30°. Point of insertion is 2–3 cm cranial to cricoids cartilage.

12. (a) T   (b) F   (c) T   (d) F   (e) T

Borgeat technique involves the interscalene groove. A line is drawn along interscalene groove. Point of needle insertion lies 3–5 mm below cricoid cartilage on this line. Needle is advanced caudally with slight lateral or medial angulation.

13. (a) T   (b) F   (c) T   (d) T   (e) T

The block is done in sitting position with neck flexed. The puncture point is 3 cm lateral to a midpoint of a line joining the spines of C5–C6. Ipsilateral phrenic nerve is blocked in 100 % of patients.

14. (a) F   (b) T   (c) F   (d) T   (e) T

Local twitch means needle is anterior and medial to brachial plexus. Pectoralis muscle twitch means stimulation of C4/5. Twitch of scapula is seen when needle position is posterior or deep to brachial plexus. Needle should be withdrawn and inserted more anteriorly.

15. (a) T   (b) F   (c) T   (d) T   (e) T

Needle is inserted at a lower angle to facilitate catheter positioning.

16. (a) T   (b) F   (c) F   (d) T   (e) F

Phrenic nerve palsy is seen in almost 100 % of patients with interscalene block. The incidence of hoarseness is 10–20 %. There is 15–30 % incidence of bradycardia and hypotension which is favoured by sitting position and prevented by avoiding hypovolaemia. Modified lateral technique is as described by Borgeat and is better for inserting catheters. Horner's syndrome consists of enophthalmos, ptosis and hyperaemia of conjunctiva and nasal congestion (Guttman's sign).

17. (a) F (b) T (c) F (d) T (e) T

    Pulsatile effect of subclavian artery pushes the lower trunk away, and so it is essential to inject near the nerve roots.

18. (a) T (b) F (c) T (d) T (e) T

    Point of insertion is 2 cm above insertion of sternocleidomastoid. Success rate has been shown to be unaffected by reducing the nerve stimulation to 0.5 mA or less.

19. (a) F (b) F (c) T (d) T (e)F

    The incidence is 50 % as compared to 100 % seen in interscalene block. The incidence of pneumothorax is 6.1 %. Pneumothorax can be seen as late as 12 h.

20. (a) T (b) F (c) T (d) F (e) F

    Coagulopathy is a relative contraindication as artery is nearby and can be punctured. Block is at the level of the cords. Cords surround axillary artery.

21. (a) T (b) T (c) F (d) F (e) T

    Posterior cord is in middle while medial is the deepest. Median nerve is contributed by both cords. Musculocutaneous nerve lies outside plexus.

22. (a) T (b) F (c) T (d) T (e) F

    Lateral cord lies lateral to axillary artery. Anterior divisions of lower trunk form medial cord. Posterior cord is formed from posterior divisions of C5–T1. Other terminal branches of brachial plexus are musculocutaneous nerve, median, ulnar and radial nerve. Axillary nerve supplies deltoid and teres minor.

23. (a) F   (b) F   (c) F   (d) F   (e) F

    Lateral cord innervates flexor muscles of forearm. It innervates thenar muscles and provides sensory innervations to thumb. On stimulation, flexion of fingers and flexion and opposition of thumb is seen. Musculocutaneous nerve is purely motor above elbow and purely sensory below elbow. Stimulation of musculocutaneous nerve is not a reliable indicator as it is outside the plexus, but close to cord.

24. (a) T   (b) T   (c) F   (d) T   (e) T

    Posterior cord lies deep or inferior to axillary artery.

25. (a) T   (b) F   (c) F   (d) F   (e) F

    Ulnar nerve supplies all interossei and medial two lumbricals. Median nerve is responsible for thumb opposition and ulnar nerve causes thumb adduction. Wrist flexion could be indicator of median or lateral nerve.

26. (a) T   (b) F   (c) T   (d) F   (e) T

    The insertion point is 2.5–3 cm above line. It is usually done in dorsal recumbent position with head turned towards side opposite to the block.

27. (a) T   (b) F   (c) F   (d) T   (e) F

    Needle is inserted just under the clavicle and perpendicular to the skin. The needle should be inserted lateral and not more than 6 cm. 50-mm needle should be used.

28. (a) T   (b) F   (c) F   (d) F

    Needle is inserted at an angle of 90°. Once the needle tip hits the coracoid process tip, withdraw and aim for underneath the coracoid process. Plexus is encountered at 5–6 cm.

29. (a) T   (b) T   (c) T   (d) T   (e) T

30. (a) T   (b) T   (c) T   (d) F   (e) F

31. (a) F   (b) T   (c) F   (d) T   (e) T

    Musculocutaneous and axillary nerves leave early at the level of coracoid process. Midhumeral approach is used for musculocutaneous and radial nerve.

32. (a) T   (b) T   (c) F   (d) F   (e) T

    Coracobrachialis forms the upper end of the landmark. Triple injection is the fastest way to achieve blockade. Elbow flexion indicates needle is outside neurovascular sheath; redirect needle downward and superficially. Extension of wrist and hand indicates stimulation of the radial nerve which lies below the artery.

33. (a) T   (b) F   (c) T   (d) T   (e) T

    Median nerve stimulation will cause forearm pronation. The first injection in double-injection technique is below coracobrachialis muscle, and second injection is above triceps muscle. The success rate increases with two separate injections. Transarterial technique is done as high up as in axilla. Needle should traverse artery at an oblique angle. It reduces the risk of making injection behind the artery intramuscular.

34. (a) F   (b) T   (c) T   (d) F   (e) F

    The two terminal nerves are blocked above and below the humeral bone. The risk of neurologic complications is less because of the distance between the nerves. Infraclavicular block is better than the axillary block for elbow surgery.

35. (a) F   (b) F   (c) T   (d) T   (e) F

    Toxicity manifests within 5–30 min. Symptoms of nerve damage appear within a day. Most nerve injuries are

neuropraxias and heal within a few weeks. Nerve
stimulation <0.2 mA may mean needle is intraneural.

36. (a) T   (b) T   (c) T   (d) F   (e) T

The patient lies supine with arm rotated overhead and
elbow bent to 90°. Medial epicondyle of humerus and
olecranon is palpated. Ulnar nerve runs in the groove of
the ulnar nerve at a depth of 0.5–1 cm. Paraesthesias are
elicited for injection, and fan-shaped injections are done.
Ulnar nerve supplies medial two and half fingers in
hand.

37. (a) F   (b) F   (c) T   (d) F   (e) F

Radial nerve supplies anatomical snuff box. Hypothenar
muscles are supplied by ulnar nerve. Median nerve
supplies lateral two lumbricals, while ulnar nerve
supplies all the interossei. Radial nerve is lateral to radial
artery.

38. (a) F   (b) T   (c) T   (d) T   (e) T

Superficial branches of radial nerve lie over anatomical
snuff box. Median nerve lies lateral to palmaris longus.
Flexor carpi ulnaris lies superficial to ulnar nerve. Radial
nerve is a field block because of less predictable anatomy.

Anatomical relations at wrist

39. (a) T   (b) T   (c) F   (d) T   (e) T

Radial nerve injection at wrist is a subcutaneous
injection above radial styloid. Block of dorsal sensory
branch is important which is done by inserting the
needle 1 cm proximal to radial styloid.

40. (a) F   (b) T   (c) T   (d) T

Ulnar nerve lies medial to flexor carpi ulnaris.

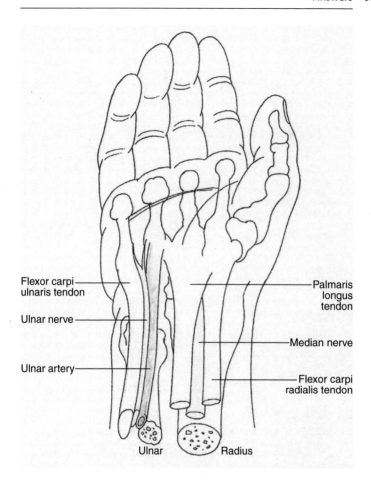

Flexor carpi
ulnaris tendon

Ulnar nerve

Ulnar artery

Palmaris
longus
tendon

Median nerve

Flexor carpi
radialis tendon

Ulnar   Radius

41. (a) F   (b) F   (c) F   (d) F   (e) T

Median nerve is blocked by inserting needle between
palmaris longus and flexor carpi radialis. Contact with
bone is more appropriate indicator of needle position.
Pronation is seen higher up in elbow stimulation.
Epinephrine is contraindicated in digital nerve blocks.

42. (a) T   (b) T   (c) F   (d) T   (e) T

Needle is inserted at an angle of 45°.

43. (a) T   (b) F   (c) T   (d) F   (e) F

It can be used as an adjunct to cervical plexus block. A single injection is given at the posterior border at mid-belly of the muscle. Complications include external jugular vein puncture.

44. (a) T   (b) T   (c) F   (d) T   (e) T

The suprascapular nerve innervates 70 % of posterior superior shoulder and acromioclavicular joint. Pneumothorax is avoided by directing needle in a caudal direction.

45. (a) T   (b) F   (c) F   (d) T   (e) T

The nerve supplies supraspinatus and infraspinatus muscles and shoulder and acromioclavicular joints. The optimum position is sitting with the neck tilted forwards. The landmarks are spine of scapula and acromion.

46. (a) T   (b) F   (c) T   (d) T   (e) T

The block only decreases the cutaneous sensation associated with the tourniquet. Complications are rare because of superior placement of the block.

47. (a) T   (b) F   (c) F   (d) T   (e) T

Intravenous regional anaesthesia can be done as an outpatient's procedure. Two intravenous access points are required, one in each extremity. The pressure in the cuff should be 80–100 mmHg more than the patient's systolic pressure. The rate of injection should not be more than 20 ml/min. Intermittent deflation over a period of 10 min with complete inflation in between should be done to avoid toxicity.

48. (a) T   (b) T   (c) T   (d) F   (e) T

Local anaesthetics with vasoconstrictor action should be used. Prilocaine 0.5 % (3–4 mg/kg) can be used and has the best ratio between anaesthetic potency and toxicity. Other agents that can be used are mepivacaine 0.5 % or lidocaine 0.5 % (1.5–3 mg/kg). The onset time is 5–10 min. The maximum operating time for the block is 1 h.

	Interscalene block	Infraclavicular block	Axillary block
Advantages	Clear anatomical landmarks	No special position required	Clear anatomical landmarks
	Patient cooperation not required	More favourable distribution of local anaesthetic	Can be used as continuous block
	Dense block extending to cervical components	Catheter easy to maintain	Safe for anaesthesia of hand and arm
	Surgery is possible in arm and shoulder	No respiratory complications	
	The risk of pneumothorax is low		
Disadvantages	Necessary to produce paraesthesias in landmark technique	Pneumothorax	Shoulder and upper arm surgery cannot be performed
	Ulnar nerve may be missed	Vascular placement	Musculocutaneous nerve and axillary nerve may be missed

5 Lower Limb Blocks

1. Lower limb neurological assessment:
   (a) Plantar flexion is aided by sciatic nerve.
   (b) Obturator nerve assessment is a robust indicator of sacral plexus.
   (c) Lateral femoral cutaneous can be assessed by eliciting eversion of foot.
   (d) Femoral branch supplies skin on the medial aspect of the feet.
   (e) Earliest sign of femoral nerve block is loss of quadriceps motor power.

2. Lumbar plexus:
   (a) Block is sufficient on its own for major surgery of lower extremity.
   (b) Plexus is derived from L234 which is surrounded by psoas major muscle.
   (c) Femoral division is formed by anterior division of L234.
   (d) Lateral femoral cutaneous and genitofemoral nerve are purely cutaneous.
   (e) Obturator nerve sends motor branches to adductors.

3. Lumbar plexus block:
   (a) Iliac crest and spines form landmark.
   (b) Local twitch of paravertebral muscles is a confirmatory sign.
   (c) Successful block depends on dispersion of local anaesthetic in the fascial plane.

R. Gupta, D. Patel, *Multiple Choice Questions in Regional Anaesthesia*,
DOI 10.1007/978-3-642-31257-1_5, © Springer-Verlag Berlin Heidelberg 2013

(d) Motor stimulation with low current may indicate placement of needle inside the dural sheath.

(e) Twitches of hamstring muscles can be seen.

4. Psoas compartment block:
   (a) Represents cranial and dorsal paravertebral access to lumbar plexus.
   (b) Is as good as "3-in-1 block".
   (c) Loss of resistance is seen due to penetration of fascial compartment between quadrates lumborum and psoas major muscle.
   (d) Post injection pain may be seen.
   (e) Subarachnoid or epidural injection may be seen.

5. Lumbar plexus block:
   (a) Psoas muscle stimulation is manifested as flexion of thigh.
   (b) Tuohy needle is preferable for continuous block.
   (c) Breakthrough pain on continuous infusion is best managed by increasing the rate of infusion.
   (d) Systemic toxicity is more often seen.
   (e) Local anaesthetic spread to epidural space is rarely seen.

6. Obturator nerve block:
   (a) Useful in relief of adductor muscle spasm.
   (b) Useful in suppressing obturator reflex in TURP.
   (c) Can be used in chronic pain management.
   (d) Inguinal lymphadenopathy is a contraindication for the block.
   (e) Obturator neuropathy is a relative contraindication.

7. Obturator nerve:
   (a) Is purely motor.
   (b) Is derived from anterior primary rami L234.
   (c) Is separated from femoral nerve by iliopsoas muscle.
   (d) Innervates hip joint.
   (e) It innervates visceral peritoneum.

8. Obturator nerve:
    (a) Divides into anterior and posterior branch in obturator foramen.
    (b) Innervates femoral artery.
    (c) Forms subsartorial plexus with sciatic nerve.
    (d) Does not innervate knee joint.
    (e) Paralysis leads to a total loss of adduction.

9. Obturator nerve:
    (a) May branch well after reaching thigh.
    (b) Sensory cutaneous branch is often absent.
    (c) Accessory obturator nerve is seen in majority of patients.
    (d) Supplies only adductors.
    (e) Posterior branch descends between adductor brevis in front and adductor magnus behind.

10. Obturator nerve block (3-in-1 block):
    (a) Posterior superior iliac spine forms a landmark.
    (b) 3-in-1 block entails large volumes of local anaesthetic under fascia iliaca.
    (c) Distal compression helps in increasing efficacy.
    (d) Increase in volume helps in spread of 3-in-1 block.
    (e) Catheters if placed have a high rate of success.

11. Obturator nerve block:
    (a) Iliofascial approach is better than 3-in-1 block in adults.
    (b) Iliofascial approach may spare obturator nerve.
    (c) Psoas compartment block is more reliable for obturator nerve blockade.
    (d) Parasacral approach provides more consistent anaesthetic of all branches of sciatic nerve.
    (e) Labat's classic technique is most popular approach.

12. Obturator nerve block (Labat's technique):
    (a) Patient position is prone.
    (b) Limb should be abducted to 30°.
    (c) The tip of needle should be on top of the obturator tendon.
    (d) Contraction of thigh adductor muscles can be seen.

13. Obturator nerve block (perivascular inguinal block):
    (a) Selective block of two branches of obturator nerve is done.
    (b) Femoral artery and tendon of adductor muscle at the pubic tubercle are the landmarks.
    (c) Needle is inserted at midpoint of a line between pulse of femoral artery and tendon of long adductor muscle.
    (d) Higher incidence of pelvic complications.
    (e) Hip joint is blocked as well.

14. Obturator nerve block:
    (a) Sensory testing is reliable for the block.
    (b) Block manifests as reduction in adduction strength.
    (c) Sensory block is seen in a small area on posteromedial aspect of the knee.
    (d) Complications reported are rare.
    (e) Can cause visceral perforation.

15. Femoral nerve block:
    (a) Is appropriate for surgery on anterior aspect of the thigh.
    (b) Is good for post-operative analgesia after knee surgery.
    (c) Continuous blockade can reduce post-operative opioid requirements.
    (d) Previous ilioinguinal surgery is a contraindication.

16. Femoral nerve:
    (a) Is formed by ventral division of anterior rami of L234.
    (b) Emerges from inguinal ligament under fascia iliaca.

(c) Saphenous nerve is a major supply of lateral aspect of leg.

(d) Lies medial to femoral artery in inguinal crease.

(e) Anterior branch has no cutaneous sensation.

17. Femoral nerve block:

(a) Landmarks are inguinal ligament, pubic tubercle and femoral artery.

(b) Patient is in lateral position.

(c) Needle insertion is medial to the pulsation of femoral artery.

(d) Needle is inserted perpendicularly.

(e) Quadriceps muscle the contraction is the endpoint.

18. Femoral nerve block:

(a) Loss of resistance indicates needle advancement through fascia lata.

(b) Twitch of sartorius muscle indicates needle tip is anterior and medial to femoral nerve.

(c) Multiple-injection technique is better than single injection.

(d) Larger volume increases the success rate.

(e) Weakness of extension of knee is a sign of blockade.

19. Continuous femoral nerve block:

(a) Addition of clonidine helps in prolongation of analgesia.

(b) Local anaesthesia can diffuse into epidural space.

(c) Paraesthesia is a reliable sign of femoral nerve stimulation.

(d) Catheter placement >5 days is an advantage.

(e) There is a high incidence of nerve injury.

20. 3-in-1 block:

(a) Can be used for various surgeries.

(b) Femoro-popliteal bypass graft is a relative contraindication.

(c) Lateral femoral cutaneous nerve is purely sensory.
(d) More proximal parts of thigh are better blocked than distal parts.
(e) Obturator nerve block is not important as there is no sensory distribution.

21. 3-in-1 block:
  (a) Anterior-superior iliac spine is a landmark.
  (b) Patient position is supine with both legs extended.
  (c) Patellar twitch at 0.3 mA is accepted as an endpoint.
  (d) High-frequency linear ultrasound probe is required.
  (e) Anterior branch of obturator nerve is easily visualised under ultrasound.

22. 3-in-1 block:
  (a) Femoral artery serves as one of the landmarks.
  (b) Dancing patella is the endpoint.
  (c) Compression of the area should be done after extension of leg.
  (d) Unexpected long nerve block may indicate nerve injury.
  (e) Catheter can be inserted for infusions.

23. Sciatic nerve:
  (a) Is the largest terminal branch of lumbosacral plexus
  (b) Exits pelvis above piriformis muscle.
  (c) Division occurs distal to femur.
  (d) Supplies hip joint.
  (e) Long head of biceps crosses sciatic nerve obliquely.

24. Sacral plexus:
  (a) Is formed by S1–S3 roots.
  (b) The roots combine to form sciatic nerve on the dorsal surface of piriformis.

    (c) Common peroneal and tibial nerves are separated right from onset.

    (d) Common peroneal nerve passes above the piriformis and tibial nerve below it.

    (e) Large volume is required to block sciatic nerve because of large size.

25. Sciatic nerve block:

    (a) Provides complete anaesthesia of leg below the knee.

    (b) Greater trochanter is one of the landmarks.

    (c) Needle insertion is 4 cm distal to line connecting greater trochanter and posterior superior iliac spine.

    (d) Needle is inserted perpendicularly to the skin.

    (e) Cephalad angulation helps in identifying nerve.

26. Sciatic nerve block (perisacral approach):

    (a) Posterior superior iliac spine is a landmark.

    (b) Needle insertion point is 6 cm caudal to line joining posterior superior iliac spine and inferior trochanter.

    (c) Twitches of hamstrings are acceptable.

    (d) Responses to both tibial nerve and common peroneal nerve should be seen before injecting.

    (e) Is less time consuming as compared to Winnie's approach.

27. Sciatic nerve block (anterior approach):

    (a) Is suitable for hip surgery.

    (b) Best suited for people who cannot be positioned in the lateral position.

    (c) Catheter insertion is easy.

    (d) Needle insertion point is marked 4–5 cm distally on the line connecting femoral artery and perpendicular femoral crease.

    (e) Bone contact is required for the block.

28. Sciatic nerve (popliteal region):
    (a) Tibial nerve passes between two heads of the gastrocnemius muscle.
    (b) Tibial nerve divides near lateral malleolus.
    (c) Common peroneal nerve divides after entering peroneus longus muscle.
    (d) Common peroneal nerve supplies knee joint capsule.
    (e) Saphenous nerve is the terminal branch of tibial nerve.

29. Sciatic nerve block (popliteal approach):
    (a) Suitable for foot and ankle surgery.
    (b) Has the same duration of effect as ankle block.
    (c) Short vein stripping can be done under it.
    (d) Knee flexion is lost as part of the block.
    (e) Calf tourniquet can be used under this block.

30. Sciatic nerve:
    (a) Common peroneal nerve supplies knee joint.
    (b) Sural nerve is the terminal branch of tibial nerve.
    (c) Tibial nerve supplies ankle joint.
    (d) Usually divides after traversing popliteal crease.
    (e) Popliteal artery and vein lie medial to nerve is popliteal fossa.

31. Sciatic nerve block (intertendinous approach):
    (a) Popliteal fossa crease is one of the landmarks.
    (b) Insertion of needle is midpoint between tendons.
    (c) Local muscular twitches should not be seen if needle is in midline.
    (d) Popliteal nerve stimulation is manifested as dorsiflexion.
    (e) Tibial nerve stimulation causes inversion.

32. Sciatic nerve block (lateral approach):
    (a) Can be done in supine position.
    (b) Sciatic nerve is encountered between biceps and semitendinosus.
    (c) Stimulation of tibial nerve is encountered first.
    (d) Needle insertion is between vastus lateralis and biceps femoris muscle.
    (e) Flexing patient's leg helps in identification of the popliteal fossa crease.

33. Nerves at ankle:
    (a) Tibial nerve divides into medial and lateral plantar nerves.
    (b) Common peroneal nerve runs through peroneus longus muscle.
    (c) Deep peroneal nerve passes with dorsalis pedis artery into the first interosseous space.
    (d) Sural nerve is formed by medial sural cutaneous nerve and peroneal-communicating branch.
    (e) Saphenous nerve ends at the level of big toe.

34. Ankle block:
    (a) Prolonged analgesia can be achieved without affecting motor power.
    (b) Can be used for diagnosis of chronic pain.
    (c) Four nerves need to be blocked for effective analgesia.
    (d) Plantar aspect is supplied by medial and lateral plantar nerves.
    (e) The posterior tibial nerve can be blocked in front of medial malleolus.

35. Ankle block:
    (a) Extensor hallucis longus is one of the landmarks.
    (b) Saphenous, sural and superficial nerves are all blocked by circumferential injection near malleoli.

(c) Deep peroneal nerve can be blocked just medial to extensor hallucis longus.
(d) Posterior tibial nerve is blocked by injecting posterior to posterior tibial nerve.
(e) Deep peroneal nerve is blocked medial to dorsalis pedis artery.

36. Lateral femoral cutaneous nerve block:
    (a) Can be used in small vein graft surgery and is diagnostic for meralgia paraesthetica.
    (b) Cutaneous supply is to anterior lateral aspect of the thigh.
    (c) Posterior superior iliac spine is an important landmark.
    (d) Contributes to patellar plexus.
    (e) Needle gives a loss of resistance through fascia lata.

37. Lateral femoral cutaneous nerve block:
    (a) Nerve arises from L345.
    (b) Helps in tourniquet pain.
    (c) Loss of resistance is seen with penetration of fascia lata.
    (d) Paraesthesias are elicited after needle insertion.
    (e) Long needles are required.

38. Saphenous nerve:
    (a) Is a mixed nerve.
    (b) Is a component of adductor canal.
    (c) Follows saphenous vein down to the leg.
    (d) Has a connection with superficial peroneal nerve.
    (e) Supplies medial side of tibia and medial calf skin.

39. Saphenous nerve block:
    (a) Terminal branch of sciatic nerve.
    (b) Innervates medial aspect of lower leg up to the first metatarsophalangeal joint.

(c) Usually blocked by subcutaneous infiltration around tibial tuberosity.

(d) Paravenous technique involves infiltration around saphenous nerve.

(e) Transsartorial approach is most effective for the blockade.

40. Sural nerve:

(a) Blockade can be used for lateral aspect of ankle and feet.

(b) Is a branch of common peroneal nerve.

(c) Passes between lateral malleolus and calcaneus.

(d) Landmarks for blockade are Achilles tendon and lateral malleolus.

(e) Is joined by a branch of common peroneal nerve to supply the area.

Answers

1. (a) T   (b) F   (c) F   (d) T   (e) F

   Obturator nerve assessment is a robust indicator of
   lumbar plexus. Lateral cutaneous femoral nerve is purely
   sensory nerve and is assessed by a pinch on proximal
   lateral thigh. Saphenous is a branch of the femoral nerve
   that supplies the medial aspect of feet. Earliest sign of
   femoral nerve block is loss of temperature discrimination
   in saphenous nerve territory.

2. (a) F   (b) T   (c) F   (d) T   (e) T

   Sciatic nerve needs to be blocked as well for any surgery
   on lower extremity. Femoral nerve is formed by posterior
   rami of L234, while anterior rami form obturator nerve.

3. (a) T   (b) F   (c) T   (d) T   (e) T

   Quadriceps stimulation is confirmatory sign of lumbar
   plexus. Motor stimulation with current less than 0.5 mA
   should not be used. Hamstring twitches may be seen when
   the needle is inserted too far in, causing stimulation of
   sciatic plexus.

4. (a) T   (b) T   (c) T   (d) T   (e) T

   Adequate block can be as good as "3-in-1 block". The pain
   may increase after the block due to spasm in paravertebral
   region.

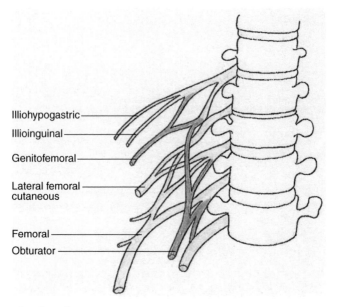

Lumbar plexus

5. (a) T   (b) T   (c) F   (d) T   (e) F

Psoas muscle stimulation is seen when needle is inserted too deep. Breakthrough pain is managed by giving a bolus. Systemic toxicity is seen because of large muscle beds providing large vascular area for local anaesthetic absorption. Local anaesthetic spread is seen in up to 15 % of cases.

6. (a) T   (b) T   (c) T   (d) T   (e) F

There is a direct stimulation seen in TURP which causes sudden violent adductor muscle spasm. This can lead to bladder wall perforation, vessel laceration, incomplete tumour resection and haematoma. Obturator neuropathy is a relative contraindication.

7. (a) F (b) T (c) T (d) T (e) F

Obturator nerve is a mixed nerve which provides cutaneous sensation behind knee. It innervates parietal peritoneum.

8. (a) T (b) T (c) F (d) T (e) F

Obturator nerve divides mostly after leaving the foramen, but in a few may divide in the canal. Subsartorial plexus is formed by obturator nerve and femoral nerve. The plexus supplies sensory branches to posteromedial aspect of inferior one third of thigh. Anterior branch contributes to capsule of hip joint. Adductor magnus fibres get nerve supply from sciatic nerve also, so obturator palsy will not cause paralysis on its own.

9. (a) T (b) T (c) F (d) F (e) T

In 15 % of patients, obturator nerve branches after reaching thigh. Accessory obturator nerve is seen in 20 % of patients. It also supplies gracilis which causes knee flexion and obturator externus which causes lateral rotation of thigh.

10. (a) F (b) T (c) F (d) F (e) F

The landmarks are pubic tubercle, anterior-superior iliac spine, femoral artery and tendon of long adductor muscle. Catheters do not increase success rate as only 23 % are reliably placed.

11. (a) F (b) T (c) T (d) T (e) T

Iliofascial approach is better for blocking lateral femoral cutaneous nerve.

12. (a) F   (b) T   (c) T   (d) T

13. (a) T   (b) T   (c) T   (d) F   (e) F
    Both anterior and posterior branches need to be blocked.
    Pelvic complications are less as insertion point is away
    from intrapelvic contents. Articular branches are not
    blocked.

14. (a) F   (b) T   (c) T   (d) T   (e) T
    Sensory testing is reliable because of variability in
    sensory distribution.

15. (a) T   (b) T   (c) T   (d) T
    Femoral nerve block is good for 8–12 h post-operatively
    for analgesia. Contraindications include previous
    ilioinguinal lymphadenopathy, local infections, perineal
    infections and femoral neuropathy.

16. (a) F   (b) T   (c) F   (d) F   (e) F
    It is formed by dorsal divisions of L234. Saphenous
    branch supplies medial side of feet. Femoral nerve lies
    lateral to the femoral artery. Anterior branch supplies
    skin of the anterior and medial aspect of the thigh.

17. (a) F   (b) F   (c) F   (d) F   (e) T
    The landmarks for the block are inguinal ligament,
    inguinal crease and femoral artery. The position is
    supine with extremity abducted to 10–20°. Needle
    insertion is lateral to femoral artery below inguinal
    crease. Needle is inserted at an angle of 45°. The
    endpoint is patellar twitch.

18. (a) T   (b) T   (c) T   (d) F   (e) T

19. (a) F   (b) T   (c) F   (d) F   (e) F

Addition of clonidine delays motor block. Catheters should not be left for more than 72 h as after this time there is a risk of bacterial colonisation. The incidence of nerve injury is 0.25 %.

20. (a) T   (b) T   (c) T   (d) F   (e) F

The "3-in-1" block is an infero-anterior approach to the femoral nerve, lateral femoral cutaneous nerve and obturator nerve. The block can be used for patellar surgeries, hip fracture surgeries and femoral shaft surgeries. More proximal parts of thigh are innervated by sensory nerves from abdominal wall.

21. (a) T   (b) T   (c) T   (d) T   (e) F

The leg to be blocked is laterally rotated by 15–20°. Higher-frequency probe is required because of superficial position of femoral nerve. Anterior branch is difficult to visualise because of its location between adductor brevis and adductor longus.

22. (a) T   (b) T   (c) F   (d) T   (e) T

Femoral artery is palpated 1–2 cm distal to the inguinal ligament. The injection point lies about 1–1.5 cm lateral to the pulsation. After the injection, compression massage of the injection area is carried out and thigh is flexed for 1 min. Unexpected prolonged block could be because of intraneural injection.

23. (a) T   (b) F   (c) F   (d) T   (e) T

Sciatic nerve exits under piriformis and its division occur proximally to femur.

24. (a) F   (b) F   (c) F   (d) T   (e) F

    The sacral plexus is formed by L4 to S3. The ventral roots converge to form sciatic nerve. Only in 15 % the two nerves are separated at the outset.

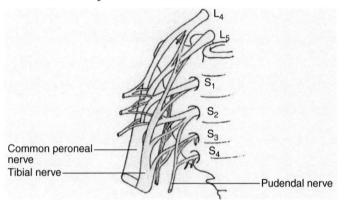

    Fig: Sacral plexus

25. (a) F   (b) T   (c) T   (d) T   (e) T

    It provides complete anaesthesia of medial strip of the skin. Other landmark is posterior superior iliac spine.

26. (a) T   (b) T   (c) T   (d) F   (e) T

    Other landmark is ischial tuberosity. Twitches to hamstrings are accepted as block is proximal, and nerves are still not divided. Response to either tibial or common peroneal nerve is sufficient.

27. (a) F   (b) T   (c) F   (d) T   (e) F

    The block is suitable for the operations below the knee. Catheter insertion is easy because of perpendicular position. Bone contact is usually the lesser trochanter. The feet should be moved laterally which takes the trochanter out of the way.

28. (a) T   (b) F   (c) F   (d) T   (e) F

Tibial nerve runs distally together with the posterior tibial artery though the calf musculature, as far as the midpoint between the medial malleolus and the calcaneus to medial side of foot joint. Common peroneal nerve divides into mainly sensory superficial peroneal nerve and motor deep peroneal nerve before entering peroneus longus muscle. Saphenous nerve is the terminal branch of femoral nerve.

29. (a) T   (b) F   (c) T   (d) F   (e) T

Ankle block is less in duration as compared to lower extremity block.

30. (a) T   (b) F   (c) T   (d) F   (e) T

Sciatic nerve usually divides before popliteal crease.

31. (a) T   (b) T   (c) T   (d) F   (e) T

The landmarks are popliteal fossa crease, tendon of biceps femoris and semitendinosus and semimembranosus medially. Popliteal nerve stimulation is manifested as plantar flexion.

32. (a) T   (b) T   (c) F   (d) T   (e) T

Common peroneal nerve is positioned lateral and more superficial than the tibial nerve and is stimulated first.

33. (a) T   (b) T   (c) T   (d) T   (e) F

Saphenous nerve never reaches the big toe.

34. (a) T   (b) T   (c) F   (d) T   (e) F

Ankle block is used for diagnosis of sympathetically mediated pain. Five nerves need to be blocked—sural nerve, posterior tibial nerve, superficial peroneal nerve, deep peroneal nerve and saphenous nerve. The posterior tibial nerve can be blocked behind the medial malleolus.

35. (a) T (b) T (c) F (d) T (e) T

The landmarks are external hallucis longus, medial and lateral malleoli, Achilles tendon, posterior tibial artery, dorsalis pedis artery and sustentaculum tali.

36. (a) T (b) T (c) F (d) T (e) T

Anterior-superior iliac spine is an important landmark. Patellar plexus is formed by anterior division of femoral nerve with saphenous nerve and lateral femoral cutaneous nerve.

37. (a) F (b) T (c) T (d) F (e) F

The nerve is formed by L23. Paraesthesias are not elicited but a fan-shaped injection of local anaesthetic is carried out.

38. (a) F (b) T (c) T (d) T (e) T

The nerve is purely sensory. Other contents of adductor canal are femoral artery, saphenous vein and nerve to vastus medialis.

39. (a) F (b) T (c) T (d) T (e) T

It is a terminal branch of femoral nerve.

40. (a) T (b) F (c) T (d) T (e) T

Sural nerve is a branch of tibial nerve. Skin wheal is raised lateral to Achilles tendon just above medial malleolus.

6 Ophthalmic Block

1. Orbit:
   (a) Approximate volume is 30 ml.
   (b) Mean average axial length of eyeball is 23.5 cm.
   (c) Eyeball is oriented towards floor and medial wall.
   (d) Medial needle insertion puts inferior oblique and inferior rectus at risk.
   (e) Superonasal quadrant is ideal for inserting needles.

2. Physiology of the eye:
   (a) The intraocular pressure is between 5 and 10 mmHg.
   (b) Intraocular pressure increases during coughing, physical exertion and vomiting.
   (c) Anaesthetics have no effect on intraocular pressure.
   (d) Aqueous humour is formed at the rate of 2.5 μl/min.
   (e) Ketamine increases the intraocular pressure.

3. Tenon's capsule:
   (a) Covers both globe and extracellular muscles.
   (b) Blends with the connective tissue of extraocular muscles.
   (c) Is penetrated Penetrated by rectus muscles.
   (d) Conjunctiva is fused with tenon's capsule.
   (e) Is pierced Pierced by ciliary nerves and vessels.

4. Ophthalmic block:
   (a) Smaller needles give better tactile information and are less likely to damage intraorbital structures.
   (b) Curved needles are better than straight needles.

R. Gupta, D. Patel, *Multiple Choice Questions in Regional Anaesthesia*,
DOI 10.1007/978-3-642-31257-1_6, © Springer-Verlag Berlin Heidelberg 2013

(c) Blunt-tip needles help in avoiding puncture in patients with long eyes.

(d) Retrobulbar block involves administering local anaesthetic into muscle cone.

5. Pre-assessment for ophthalmic anaesthesia:
   (a) Starvation is necessary for nerve blocks
   (b) All medications should be stopped before the blocks.
   (c) Anticoagulant medication use is a contraindication.
   (d) Antibiotics should be given for patients with heart disease.
   (e) Axial length of eyeball should be known before the block.

6. Retrobulbar block:
   (a) Gaze should be upwards and inwards for the block.
   (b) Large volumes of local anaesthetic are required for the block.
   (c) Orbicularis oculi is not blocked.
   (d) Low incidence of complications.
   (e) Brainstem anaesthesia can occur.

7. Complications associated with retrobulbar block:
   (a) Blindness.
   (b) Chemosis.
   (c) Perforation of eyeball.
   (d) Subarachnoid injection.
   (e) Oculocardiac reflex.

8. Peribulbar block:
   (a) Needle inserted into extra conal place.
   (b) Requires large volumes of local anaesthetic.
   (c) Orbicularis oculi is not blocked.
   (d) Double Two-injection technique is better than single-injection technique.
   (e) Amaurosis is not seen.

9. Complications seen with peribulbar block:
    (a) Injury to trochlea and superior oblique muscles.
    (b) Higher failure rate.
    (c) Perforation of eyeball.
    (d) Eyelid haemorrhage.
    (e) Eyelid ecchymosis.

10. Combined retrobulbar and peribulbar block:
    (a) Two injections are made, one each into intraconal and extraconal space.
    (b) Transcutaneous approach is easier in patients with short palpebral fissure.
    (c) Needle is inserted diagonally, posteromedially.
    (d) Glove movement indicates that needle is in touch with sclera.
    (e) Medial gaze puts patient's optic nerve at risk.

11. Sub-tenon's block:
    (a) Involves surface anaesthesia before block.
    (b) Access through inferonasal quadrant is the most common.
    (c) Dissection involves a cut into the conjunctiva alone.
    (d) Cannula insertion may be difficult in those with medial rectus surgery.
    (e) High risk of rupture in myopes.

12. Sub-tenon's block:
    (a) Ophthalmic cannula can be plastic or metal.
    (b) Polyethylene catheter can be inserted for prolonged surgeries.
    (c) Large volumes are required to produce akinesia.
    (d) Scleral perforation is a known complication.
    (e) pH overcorrection of local anaesthetic may cause precipitation and inadequate blockade.

13. Orbit:
    (a) Superior oblique is supplied by trochlear nerve.
    (b) Lateral rectus has a separate nerve supply.
    (c) All the nerves supplying orbit and muscles have intraorbital course.
    (d) Episcleral space can be used for nerve blocks.
    (e) Extraconal space is a virtual space.

14. Peribulbar blocks:
    (a) Needle insertion through superior nasal site should be avoided.
    (b) Needle depth should be limited to 2.5 cm.
    (c) Complication rate is low.
    (d) Compression has been shown to enhance block.
    (e) Block is predictable.

15. Opthalmic block:
    (a) Mobile eye predisposes to perforation of globe.
    (b) Retrobulbar haemorrhage can manifest as subconjunctival ecchymosis.
    (c) Internal carotid artery injection has been seen with retrobulbar anaesthesia.
    (d) Optic nerve sheath injection may present as ptosis.
    (e) Muscle palsy can be seen.

16. Oculocardiac reflex:
    (a) Tachycardia is seen.
    (b) Afferent pathway is trigeminal and efferent is vagus.
    (c) Asystole can occur.
    (d) Mostly seen in elderly.
    (e) Prophylaxis of atropine in adults not required.

17. Eye blocks (complications):
    (a) Seizures may be seen.
    (b) Globe perforation and rupture has good prognosis.

   (c) High myopes are more susceptible to perforation.

   (d) Venous puncture can lead to compressive haematoma.

   (e) Sub-tenon is a better approach for those on anticoagulants.

18. Topical anaesthesia of eye:

   (a) Phacoemulsification can be done.

   (b) Akinesia is seen.

   (c) Intracameral injection involves injection of local anaesthetic into posterior chamber.

   (d) Intracorneal injections are risk free.

   (e) Eye drops are better than lidocaine gel.

19. Sub-tenon's block:

   (a) Larger volumes are helpful in analgesia of entire globe.

   (b) Akinesia is seen.

   (c) Chemosis is never seen.

   (d) Low risk of complications.

   (e) Surgical technique makes small incision in bulbar conjunctiva.

20. Ophthalmic blocks:

   (a) Normal axial length is 23 mm.

   (b) Staphylomas are mostly seen in superior pole.

   (c) Increase in axial length only marginally increases the risk of staphyloma.

   (d) More risk of damage if inferotemporal approach is used.

   (e) Previous history of surgery for retinal detachment or choroidal melanoma mandates general anaesthesia.

21. Ophthalmic anatomy:
    (a) Depth from orbital vein to optic foramen is 5 cm.
    (b) Superior oblique muscle is most difficult to anaesthetise.
    (c) Adjacent facial nerve block improves quality of anaesthesia.
    (d) Sensory supply of globe is via trigeminal nerve.
    (e) Both superior and inferior ophthalmic vein pass through the superior oblique fissure.

22. Modified retrobulbar block:
    (a) Needle is inserted at inferotemporal area.
    (b) Needle is directed medially and posteriorly.
    (c) Optic nerve is at risk as it lies in the medial half.
    (d) Neutral gaze is preferred.
    (e) Pressure on the globe is required for uniform distribution of local anaesthetic.

23. Orbit anatomy:
    (a) Frontal bone forms the roof.
    (b) Optic canal transmits optic nerve and ophthalmic artery.
    (c) All the nerves supplying the orbit pass through superior oblique fissure except lacrimal nerve which passes through inferior oblique fissure.
    (d) Sclera covers eyeball except over superior end.
    (e) Orbicularis oculi assists in blinking.

24. Sensory nerve supply of orbit is:
    (a) Trigeminal nerve.
    (b) Supraorbital nerve.
    (c) Lacrimal nerve.
    (d) Long ciliary nerves.
    (e) Oculomotor nerve.

25. Complications of ophthalmic block:
    (a) Injections through conjunctiva are less painful as compared to skin.
    (b) Retrobulbar haemorrhage is seen in 0.15–1.7 % of patients.
    (c) Perforation presents as hypotonia and sudden loss of vision.
    (d) Amaurosis is seen with peribulbar injection.
    (e) Subarachnoid injection is possible.

Answers

1. (a) T   (b) T   (c) F   (d) T   (e) F

   Eyeball is oriented towards roof and lateral wall.
   Superonasal quadrant is dangerous as are trochlea and
   belly of superior oblique.

2. (a) F   (b) T   (c) F   (d) T   (e) T

   Intraocular pressure is between 10 and 20 mmHg. The
   pressure is high in patients with a large-diameter eyeball,
   recumbent position, coughing, physical exertion and
   vomiting. Inhalational anaesthetics, barbiturates, opioids
   and propofol decrease the intraocular pressure, whereas
   ketamine and muscle relaxants have the opposite effect.
   The rate of synthesis is 2.5 μl/min.

3. (a) T   (b) T   (c) T   (d) T   (e) T

   Conjunctiva is fused with tenon's capsule.

4. (a) T   (b) F   (c) F   (d) T

   Straight needles are simple to use and are less expensive.
   Long eyes have exceptionally thin sclera making them
   prone to perforate.

5. (a) F   (b) F   (c) F   (d) T   (e) T

   Medications should be continued as prescribed. Diabetics
   should receive their medications. Patients on
   anticoagulation should receive either sub-tenon's block or
   topical anaesthesia.

6. (a) F   (b) F   (c) T   (d) F   (e) T

   The gaze should be neutral as moving the eyeball upwards and inwards brings the macula and needle directly in the path of needle. Small amount of local anaesthetic (1.5–4 ml) usually suffices.

7. (a) T   (b) T   (c) T   (d) T   (e) T

   Orbit is a well vascularised, and haemorrhage can lead to compartment syndrome and blindness. Retinal haemorrhage and vitreous haemorrhage can lead to loss of vision. Chemosis is seen in 25–40 % and is due to injection of larger volumes of local anaesthetics.

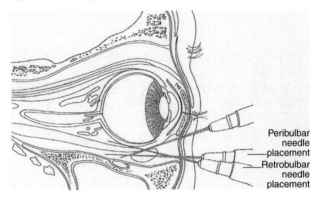

Retrobulbar and peribulbar block

8. (a) T   (b) T   (c) F   (d) F   (e) T

   Typical volumes between 6 and 10 ml are required for the block. Orbicularis oculi is blocked because of injection of large volumes. Local anaesthetic flows retrograde through orbital septum and causes paralysis.

9. (a) T   (b) T   (c) T   (d) T   (e) T

   Injuries to trochlea and superior oblique muscle can occur which can be prevented by avoiding superonasal injection.

This may lead to poorer results. The failure rate is 10–20 %. The incidence of perforation is 1:12,000–16,000.

10. (a) T   (b) T   (c) T   (d) T   (e) T

11. (a) T   (b) T   (c) F   (d) T   (e) T

Surface anaesthesia is required as it involves dissection. Most commonly used anaesthetics are amethocaine and proxymetacaine. Access through inferonasal quadrant helps avoid damage to vortex veins. The cut involves conjunctiva and tenon's capsule. Canula insertion is difficult in those with medial rectus surgery, previous detachment surgery and those with a history of pterygium. High risk of rupture in myopes is due to posterior staphyloma or sclera thinning.

12. (a) T   (b) T   (c) T   (d) T   (e) T

13. (a) T   (b) T   (c) F   (d) T   (e) T

All the nerves have intraorbital course except nerve to orbicularis oculi which has an extraorbital course.

14. (a) T   (b) T   (c) T   (d) F   (e) F

Needle insertion through superonasal site increases the risk of globe perforation and superior oblique muscle injury. Needle insertion more than 2.5 cm increases the risk of injection into retrobulbar space and injection directly into foramen. Compression lowers intraocular pressure. The main disadvantage of the block is unpredictable spread.

15. (a) T   (b) T   (c) T   (d) T   (e) T

Muscular palsy can be seen if high concentration of local anaesthetic is used, e.g. 4 % lidocaine.

16. (a) T   (b) T   (c) T   (d) F   (e) T

Mostly, bradycardia is seen because of traction on extraocular muscles. It is mostly seen in children (90 %).

17. (a) T   (b) F   (c) T   (d) F   (e) T

If local anaesthetic is injected into an artery, the blood flow can reverse to internal carotid artery and can cause seizures. Incidence of globe perforation is 1:350, and the prognosis is poor if diagnosis is delayed. High myopes are susceptible to staphyloma which increases the risk of rupture. If axial length is >26 mm, sub-tenon block is preferred. Arterial puncture can lead to compressive haematoma which can compromise retinal perfusion.

18. Topical anaesthesia of eye:
(a) T   (b) F   (c) F   (d) F   (e) F

Akinesia is not seen which may make surgery hazardous. The capacity for anterior chamber is 0.1 ml of local anaesthetic. Corneal endothelium is prone to toxicity by local anaesthetic.

19. (a) T   (b) T   (c) F   (d) T   (e) T

Large volumes of local anaesthetic always cause chemosis. Small incision is done in conjunctiva and tenon's capsule to gain access into episcleral space. Injection of low volumes of local anaesthetic is used.

20. (a) T   (b) F   (c) F   (d) T   (e) T

Staphylomas are mostly seen in posterior pole and equator. Axial length of 27–29 mm has an incidence of staphyloma of 155, and the incidence increases to 60 % with an axial length of 31 mm.

21. (a) T   (b) T   (c) F   (d) F   (e) F

Superior oblique muscle lies outside fibro-tendinous ring and difficult to anaesthetise. Globe is supplied by long- and short-ciliary nerves which are branches of ophthalmic branch of trigeminal vein. Inferior ophthalmic vein passes through inferior oblique fissure.

22. (a) T (b) T (c) T (d) T (e) T

23. (a) T (b) T (c) F (d) F (e) T

Orbit is formed of different bones. The roof is formed by frontal bone and sphenoid bone. Lateral wall is formed by zygomatic and greater wing of sphenoid. The floor is formed by maxilla, zygomatic bone and palatine bone. The medial wall is formed by ethmoid, frontal and lacrimal bone. Maxillary division of trigeminal nerve passes through inferior orbital fissure. Sclera covers eyeball except over cornea. Palpebral part of orbicularis oculi assists in blinking.

24. (a) T (b) T (c) T (d) T (e) T

Trigeminal nerve supplies sclera and cornea. Supraorbital nerve supplies superior conjunctiva and periorbital skin. The lacrimal nerve supplies lateral conjunctiva and periorbital skin. Long ciliary nerves supplied sclera and cornea and circum corneal area.

25. (a) T (b) T (c) T (d) F (e) T

Amaurosis is seen more with retrobulbar blockade of optic nerve causing temporary loss of vision. Subarachnoid injection is possible because of injection of underneath dura of optic nerve. It presents as drowsiness, vomiting and contralateral blindness.

7 Head Neck and Airway

1. Trigeminal nerve:
   - (a) Main nerve supply to lower half of face.
   - (b) Originates from Meckel's cave.
   - (c) Posterior ganglionic fibres form 3 divisions.
   - (d) Maxillary nerve exits through foramen rotundum.
   - (e) Forehead is supplied by ophthalmic nerve.

2. Mandibular nerve:
   - (a) Exits through foramen ovale.
   - (b) Supplies muscles of facial expression.
   - (c) Also supplies cutaneous sensation in front of the ear.
   - (d) Mental nerve is a terminal branch supplying chin.
   - (e) Is purely motor.

3. Trigeminal nerve block:
   - (a) Best done under fluoroscopy.
   - (b) Needle is aimed at lesser wing of sphenoid.
   - (c) Needle entry into foramen ovale is manifested as paresthesia in mandible.
   - (d) Large volumes are typically required.
   - (e) Facial numbness is seen in most patients.

4. Trigeminal block (complications):
   - (a) Total spinal anaesthesia is never seen.
   - (b) Anaesthesia dolorosa is a frequent complication.
   - (c) No ophthalmic side effects are seen.
   - (d) Pneumothorax is a known complication.
   - (e) Systemic toxicity can be seen.

R. Gupta, D. Patel, *Multiple Choice Questions in Regional Anaesthesia*,
DOI 10.1007/978-3-642-31257-1_7, © Springer-Verlag Berlin Heidelberg 2013

5. Occipital nerves:
   (a) Greater occipital nerve arises from C2.
   (b) Lies medial to occipital artery.
   (c) Lesser occipital nerve arises from second and third cervical nerve.
   (d) Lesser occipital nerve lies medial to mastoid process.
   (e) Is involved in cervicogenic headache.

6. Occipital nerve block:
   (a) Occipital protuberance forms a landmark.
   (b) Point of needle entry is in lateral one third of the line joining the landmarks.
   (c) Subcutaneous infiltration is done.
   (d) Complications are few.
   (e) 27-G needle is used.

7. Supraorbital block:
   (a) The nerve emerges from the supraorbital foramen.
   (b) The nerve supplies the lower eyelid.
   (c) Infraorbital nerve supplies maxillary incisors and canines.
   (d) The nerve is purely sensory.
   (e) Needle insertion site is in superior buccal groove.

8. Trigeminal nerve:
   (a) Has one motor root and one sensory root.
   (b) Ophthalmic branch is purely sensory.
   (c) Frontal nerve supplies conjunctiva of medial portion of the lower eyelid.
   (d) Maxillary division is purely motor.
   (e) Maxillary division supplies dura.

9. Trigeminal nerve (maxillary branch):
   (a) Is lateral to cavernous sinus.
   (b) Enters orbit through inferior orbital fissure.
   (c) Terminates as infraorbital nerve.
   (d) Supplies side of the forehead.
   (e) Forms dental plexus.

10. Ophthalmic nerve (trigeminal):
    (a) Optic branch is motor to muscles of eye.
    (b) Gives sensory fibres to oculomotor nerve, trochlear nerve and abducent nerve.
    (c) Passes through the cavernous sinus.
    (d) Passes through superior orbital fissure.
    (e) Lacrimal branch is given in the fissure.

11. Mandibular division (trigeminal):
    (a) Is both motor and sensory.
    (b) Motor nerve meets sensory nerve outside foramen ovale.
    (c) Supplies meninges and mastoid air cells.
    (d) Supplies parotid gland.
    (e) Inferior alveolar nerve provides sensation to posterior mandibular teeth.

12. Mandibular nerve block:
    (a) Otic ganglion lies on the lateral side of the nerve.
    (b) Can be used for the diagnosis of trigeminal neuralgia and glossopharyngeal neuralgia.
    (c) May cause paraesthesia in the lower jaw region.
    (d) The onset of block is most rapid in auriculotemporal nerve region.
    (e) Can cause facial paralysis.

13. Supratrochlear/supraorbital nerve block:
    (a) The nerves provide sensory innervations to forehead.
    (b) Minor operations can be done by blocking the nerves.
    (c) Supratrochlear nerve is blocked on the lateral side of nasal ala.
    (d) Haematoma formation is a complication.
    (e) Injections into supraorbital foramen should be given for effective block.

14. Infraorbital nerve block:
    (a) Can be used for the management of trigeminal neuralgia.
    (b) Can be done by extraoral and intraoral technique.
    (c) Is associated with a low risk of haematoma.
    (d) Can cause globe perforation.
    (e) Can cause nerve damage.

15. Mental nerve block:
    (a) The nerve emerges at the level of the second premolar.
    (b) The nerve supplies both the lips.
    (c) Can be used for extraction of teeth.
    (d) Injection into bony canal can cause nerve damage.
    (e) The needle is inserted at the base of the second premolar.

16. Trigeminal ganglion:
    (a) Lies on the dorsal surface of the petrous bone.
    (b) Internal carotid artery lies lateral to the ganglion.
    (c) Ganglion is enclosed in a layer of pia mater.
    (d) Ganglion is 1–2 mm in dimensions.
    (e) Is used for neurodestructive procedures for treatment of chronic pain.

17. Trigeminal ganglion block:
    (a) Increased intracranial pressure is a contraindication.
    (b) Medial edge of masseter muscle forms one of the landmarks.
    (c) Can be done without fluoroscopic guidance.
    (d) Subarachnoid injection is a possible complication.
    (e) Paraesthesia in the area of distribution of the mandibular nerve is the endpoint.

18. Stellate ganglion:
    (a) Arises from fusion of C78 with T12 ganglion.
    (b) Is developed only in 20 % of patients.
    (c) Lies dorsal to vertebral artery.
    (d) Gives off grey rami communicantes to first and
        second thoracic nerves.
    (e) Fibres also supply heart, oesophagus and trachea.

19. Stellate ganglion block:
    (a) Is helpful in patients with pain associated with
        sympathetic component.
    (b) Is helpful in Meniere's disease.
    (c) Can be done bilaterally at the same time.
    (d) Paraesthesia of the brachial plexus is the endpoint
        for injection.
    (e) Horner's sign is a sign of complete block.

20. Complications of stellate ganglion block:
    (a) Vascular complication is a common complication.
    (b) Reversible locked-in syndrome is seen.
    (c) Intrathecal injection can be prevented by repeated
        aspiration.
    (d) Bitter taste may be normally seen during the
        injection.
    (e) Bilateral block is contraindicated.

21. Superior cervical ganglion:
    (a) Arises from fusion of three or four upper cervical
        ganglia.
    (b) Has connections to middle and inferior cervical
        ganglion.
    (c) There are no known contraindications.
    (d) Lateral margin of the sternocleidomastoid forms
        one of the landmarks.
    (e) Bilateral blocks can be performed at the same time.

22. Cervical plexus block:
    (a) Is formed by upper cervical spinal nerves.
    (b) Is enough for carotid endarterectomy.
    (c) Transverse processes of C2, C3, C4 and C5 form one of the landmarks.
    (d) Endpoint is touching the groove of the transverse process.
    (e) Glossopharyngeal nerve block is one of the side effects.

23. Awake endotracheal intubation:
    (a) Oropharynx is supplied by vagus, facial and glossopharyngeal nerves.
    (b) Sensory nerve supply to anterior two thirds of tongue is by vagus nerve.
    (c) Nasal cavity is not innervated by olfactory nerve.
    (d) Oropharynx is innervated by facial, vagus and glossopharyngeal nerves.
    (e) All intrinsic laryngeal muscles are supplied by superior laryngeal nerve.

24. Airway anaesthesia:
    (a) Spraying of mucosa while inserting bronchoscope is the best method of topicalisation.
    (b) Lidocaine 0.5–4 % can be used with atomiser to anaesthetic mucosa.
    (c) Predictable anaesthesia can be achieved with topicalisation.
    (d) Phenylepinephrine has no effect on the block.

25. Glossopharyngeal blockade:
    (a) Facilitates endotracheal intubation by blocking gag reflex.
    (b) Infiltration along palatoglossal fold can help in anaesthetising the nerve.

(c) Peristyloid approach increases risk of carotid artery injection.
(d) Increases risk of toxicity.

26. Superior laryngeal nerve block:
    (a) Innervates anterior one third of the tongue.
    (b) Internal branch can be blocked lateral to greater cornu of hyoid bone.
    (c) Both internal and external branches can be blocked.
    (d) Thyrohyoid membrane puncture increases complication rate.
    (e) Aspiration of air is must before the injection.

27. Recurrent laryngeal nerve block:
    (a) Blocks vocal cords and trachea.
    (b) Best approach is transtracheal.
    (c) 1% lidocaine is infiltrated through the cricothyroid membrane.
    (d) Aspiration of free air means needle is in the larynx.
    (e) Large-gauge needle should be avoided.

28. Palatine nerves:
    (a) Supply nasal passages.
    (b) Not necessary to block for nasal fibre-optic intubation.
    (c) Pterygopalatine ganglion blockade blocks both palatine nerves.
    (d) Anaesthetic soaked cotton pledgets placed above lower turbinate blocks the pterygopalatine ganglion.
    (e) Pterygopalatine ganglion can be approached through oral cavity.

Answers

1. (a) F   (b) F   (c) T   (d) T   (e) T

Trigeminal nerve supplies the whole of the face.
Trigeminal ganglion lies in Meckel's cave which is a dural
invagination at the base of petrous portion of temporal
nerve. Posterior ganglionic fibres form ophthalmic,
maxillary and mandibular nerves. Maxillary nerve exits
through foramen rotundum, ophthalmic nerve through
superior ophthalmic fissure and mandibular through
foramen ovale.

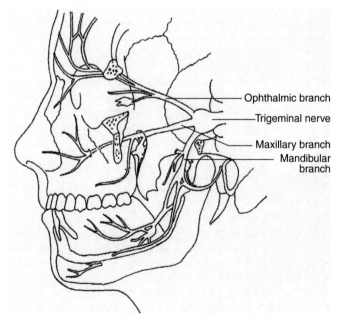

Fig: Trigeminal Nerve

2. (a) T   (b) F   (c) T   (d) T   (e) F

The nerve supplies the muscles of mastication.
Auriculotemporal nerve supplies cutaneous sensation
in front of ear.

3. (a) T   (b) F   (c) F   (d) F   (e) T

Needle is aimed at the greater wing of the sphenoid bone.
Paraesthesia is elicited in maxilla and orbit. As low as
1.0 ml can give intense analgesia.

4. (a) T   (b) T   (c) F   (d) T   (e) T

Ophthalmic side effects are seen including decreased
corneal reflex and abolition of corneal reflex and keratitis.

5. (a) T   (b) F   (c) T   (d) T   (e) T

Occipital nerve lies lateral to occipital artery.

6. (a) T   (b) F   (c) T   (d) T   (e) T

The landmark is a line joining occipital protuberance and
mastoid process. Point of needle entry is on the medial
one third of the line.

7. (a) T   (b) F   (c) T   (d) T   (e) T

Supraorbital nerve supplies lower forehead and upper
eyelid.

8. (a) T   (b) T   (c) F   (d) F   (e) T

Trigeminal nerve has a small motor branch that originates
in pons and medulla and a large sensory branch
originating from the anterior aspect of pons. Frontal
nerve supplies upper eyelid. Maxillary division is purely
sensory. Middle meningeal nerve is the only branch of
maxillary division within cranium and prevents sensory
innervations to the dura mater of middle cranial fossa.

9. (a) F (b) T (c) T (d) T (e) T

Maxillary branch of trigeminal nerve is in the lateral wall of the cavernous sinus. Zygomatic branch supplies the side of the forehead. Dental plexus is formed by three superior alveolar nerves and innervates each root of individual teeth in maxilla.

10. (a) F (b) T (c) F (d) T (e) F

The optic branch is a sensory nerve. It passes lateral to the cavernous sinus. It receives sympathetic fibres from plexus around internal carotid artery and gives fibres to the oculomotor nerve, trochlear nerve and abducent nerve. The branches given before entry into superior orbital fissure are lacrimal nerve, nasociliary nerve and frontal nerve.

11. (a) T (b) T (c) T (d) T (e) T

Motor root passes underneath the ganglion and through foramen ovale to unite with sensory root. Nervus spinosus re-enters foramen spinosum and supplies meninges and mastoid air cells. Auriculotemporal branch supplies the parotid gland.

12. (a) F (b) T (c) T (d) F (e) T

Otic ganglion lies on the medial side of the nerve after its exits through the foramen ovale. Paraesthesias are elicited in lower jaw region, lower lip and lower incisors. If the block is too superficial, facial paralysis can be seen. Other complications seen are inadvertant injections into middle meningeal and maxillary artery.

13. (a) T (b) T (c) F (d) T (e) F

The nerves supply skin of the forehead, top of the nose and skin and conjunctiva of the medial canthus. The block can be used for minor operations like of removal of cysts and atheromas. Supraorbital nerve block can be done by injecting near the supraorbital foramen. Supratrochlear nerve block can be done by injecting on the medial side of the root of the nose. The injections should not be made into the supraorbital foramen due to risk of nerve injury.

14. (a) T   (b) T   (c) F   (d) T   (e) T

The block can be used in the involvement of second division in trigeminal neuralgia. The intraoral injection is done by raising the upper lip and injecting above the second premolar tooth towards the infraorbital foramen. If the needle is inserted too far in, penetration of orbit can be seen. Temporary double vision has been noticed with the block. If injected into the bone, the block can cause nerve damage.

15. (a) T   (b) F   (c) F   (d) T   (e) T

Mental nerve exits from mental foramen at the level of the second premolar. It provides sensory nerve supply to the lower lip and chin. The technique can be used for post-dental extraction pain. The needle is inserted between the first and second premolar and into the lower reflection of the oral vestibule.

16. (a) T   (b) F   (c) F   (d) F   (e) T

The ganglion lies on dorsal surface of the petrous bone. The ganglion lies medial in the middle cranial fossa. The ganglion lies lateral to cavernous sinus, internal carotid artery and cranial nerves III–VI. The average size is 1–2 cm. The ganglion is enclosed in Meckel's cave which is a duplication of dura mater.

17. (a) T   (b) T   (c) F   (d) T   (e) T

The contraindications to the procedure are local infection, sepsis, haemorrhagic diathesis, anticoagulation treatment and significantly increased intracranial pressure. The landmarks include medial edge of masseter muscle, ipsilateral pupil and external acoustic meatus. The needle is inserted 3 cm lateral from the angle of the mouth at the level of the second molar tooth.

18. (a) T   (b) F   (c) F   (d) T   (e) T

The ganglion lies ventral to the vertebral artery. Stellate ganglion is developed in 80 % of the patients.

19. (a) T   (b) T   (c) F   (d) F   (e) F

The block is effective in Meniere's disease, sudden deafness and tinnitus. Bilateral blocks should not be done. Other contraindications include grade 2 AV block, contralateral pneumothorax, recent thrombolytic therapy, anticoagulation treatment and severe asthma/ emphysema. Horner's syndrome is not a sign of complete block. The complete cervicothoracic sympathetic block takes after 15–20 min.

20. (a) F   (b) T   (c) F   (d) F   (e) T

Vascular injection is a rare complication. The vessels at risk are vertebral artery, carotid artery, inferior thyroid artery and first intercostal artery. "Reversible locked-in syndrome" with brief apnoea and inability to move or respond to external stimuli can be seen. The patient is conscious and can move eyes vertically. Cerebrospinal fluid pressure is very low in cervical area, and the fluid is difficult to aspirate. Bitter taste may indicate rupture of the oesophagus. Bilateral blocks can lead to paresis of recurrent laryngeal nerve or phrenic nerves, both of which can be life threatening.

21. (a) T   (b) F   (c) F   (d) T   (e) F

Lingual branch of mandibular nerve supplies sensory innervations to anterior two third of tongue. Greater and lesser palatine nerves from trigeminal nerves supplies turbinates and septum. Anterior ethmoidal nerve from olfactory supplies nares and anterior one third of the septum. Superior laryngeal nerves innervates only cricothyroid where as the rest of them is supplied by recurrent laryngeal nerve.

22. (a) T   (b) F   (c) T   (d) T   (e) T

Deep cervical plexus is formed by C1 to C4 spinal nerves. Both deep and superficial cervical plexus blocks are required for carotid endarterectomy. Landmarks include posterior edge of sternocleidomastoid, caudal part of the mastoid process, Chassaignac's tubercle and transverse processes of C2, C3, C4 and C5.

23. (a) T   (b) T   (c) F   (d) F   (e) F

Superior cervical ganglion arises from 3 to 4 upper cervical ganglion. Contraindications include grade 2 AV block, recent antithrombotic therapy after myocardial infarction or pulmonary embolism, anticoagulation treatment, contralateral paresis of phrenic nerve or recurrent laryngeal nerve.

24. (a) T   (b) T   (c) F   (d) F

Topicalisation is spreading of local anaesthetic over a region of mucosa to achieve local uptake and neural blockade. It has unpredictable anaesthesia. Phenylephrine 0.5 % reduces mucosal bleeding and increases the blockade.

25. (a) T   (b) T   (c) T   (d) T

Injection is done posterior to the styloid process which is close to carotid artery.

26. (a) F   (b) T   (c) T   (d) F   (e) F

The nerve blocks base of the tongue, posterior surface of the epiglottis, aryepiglottic fold and arytenoids. Both internal and external branches can be blocked by retracting needle after contacting the hyoid bone.

Thyrohyoid membrane puncture can cause selective blockade of internal branch. Aspiration of air means laryngeal placement.

27. (a) T   (b) T   (c) F   (d) T   (e) F

4 % lidocaine is infiltrated through cricothyroid membrane. Large-gauge needles help in rapid delivery and lessen trauma due to coughing on injection.

28. (a) T   (b) F   (c) T   (d) F   (e) T

Palatine nerves are necessary to block during nasal fibre-optic intubation as they innervate nasal turbinates and posterior two thirds of the septum. Anaesthetic-soaked pledgets are placed above the upper border of the middle turbinate to posterior wall of nasopharynx. Pterygopalatine ganglion can be blocked via greater palatine foramen into pterygopalatine fossa.

8 Neuraxial Block

1. Vertebral column:
   (a) Has 33 vertebrae.
   (b) Has two curves.
   (c) Supraspinous ligament is seen as ligamentum nuchae.
   (d) Ligamentum flavum is not seen in the healthy spine.
   (e) Dural sac ends at S2 in adults.

2. Vertebral column:
   (a) Supraspinous and interspinous ligament are not traversed in paramedian approach.
   (b) Spinal cord ends at L1 at birth.
   (c) Iliac crest marks L4–L5.
   (d) T6 corresponds to umbilicus.
   (e) C8 nerve root exits above C7.

3. Sacrum:
   (a) Is formed from fusion of vertebrae.
   (b) Medial sacral crest is formed by spinous processes of upper third or fourth sacral vertebrae.
   (c) Sacral hiatus is formed by the absence of fourth and fifth arch.
   (d) Coccygeal nerve passes through the sacral hiatus.
   (e) Sacral horn represents the caudal articular process.

4. Spinal cord vessels:
   (a) Comprises of posterior artery and two anterior arteries.
   (b) Thoracolumbar segments of spinal cord gets blood supply from intercostal arteries.

R. Gupta, D. Patel, *Multiple Choice Questions in Regional Anaesthesia*,
DOI 10.1007/978-3-642-31257-1_8, © Springer-Verlag Berlin Heidelberg 2013

     (c) Median sacral arteries supply cauda equina.
     (d) Anterior spinal arteries arise from the fourth segment of the vertebral artery.
     (e) The venous plexus is in anterolateral area of the epidural space.

5. Neuraxial blocks;
     (a) Dermatomes can be innervated by multiple spinal nerves.
     (b) TURP and vaginal delivery of fetus, both need T10 block.
     (c) Lipid content of the nervous tissue is the only factor playing a role in the uptake of local anaesthetics from the subarachnoid space.
     (d) Space of Virchow-Robin assists in the uptake of local anaesthetic.
     (e) Positioning of the patient after administration of the drug does not affect the block.

6. Cerebrospinal fluid:
     (a) Is produced at 5 ml/h.
     (b) Obesity and pregnancy can increase cerebrospinal fluid.
     (c) Approximate volume in adults is 100 ml.
     (d) Production is by diffusion through epithelial cells of choroid plexus.
     (e) Lumbar CSF pressure is same in the sitting and recumbent position.

7. Local anaesthetic additives for neuraxial blockade:
     (a) Epinephrine prolongs the duration of spinal anaesthesia.
     (b) Opioids act on dorsal horn of the spinal cord.
     (c) Clonidine if injected alone intrathecally causes intense motor/sensory block.
     (d) Neostigmine administration is associated with intense nausea and vomiting.

8. Spinal anaesthesia:
   (a) Hepatic blood flow is autoregulated after spinal anaesthesia.
   (b) Renal blood flow is autoregulated after the block.
   (c) Chronic alcohol consumption increases the risk of hypotension after spinal anaesthesia.
   (d) Higher risk of bradycardia in young and healthy is seen with spinal anaesthesia.
   (e) Heart block can occur after spinal anaesthesia.

9. Unilateral spinal anaesthesia:
   (a) Blocks posterior roots only.
   (b) Reduced incidence of hypotension is seen.
   (c) Prolonged anaesthesia is seen.
   (d) Strict unilateral analgesia is achieved.
   (e) Patient needs to be on the operable site for 1 h for the full effect of anaesthesia

10. Continuous spinal anaesthesia:
    (a) Lateral decubitus position is preferred.
    (b) Repeat doses should be 30–50 % of the initial dose.
    (c) Cauda equine syndrome can be seen.
    (d) Catheter removal can be difficult.
    (e) Use of microcatheters can help reduce incidence of Post-dural puncture headache.

11. Treatment of hypotension in spinal anaesthesia:
    (a) Preloading with 500–1,500 ml is the most effective way of preventing post block hypotension.
    (b) Ephedrine works by increasing cardiac output and peripheral vascular resistance.
    (c) Reverse trendelberg should be more than 30° when hypotension is noticed.
    (d) Hypotension occurs in 33 % of non-obstetric population.
    (e) Phenylephrine can be given by infusion.

12. Bezold-Jarisch reflex:
    (a) Bradycardia, hypotension and cardiovascular collapse are seen.
    (b) Is only seen with spinal anaesthesia.
    (c) Overrides baroreceptor reflex.
    (d) Is a cardioinhibitory reflex.

13. Spinal anaesthesia:
    (a) Has no effect on lung parameters.
    (b) Dyspnoea is due to faulty gaseous exchange.
    (c) Main muscles affected are muscles of inspiration in high spinal.
    (d) Increased vagal activity is seen leading to increased peristalsis of gut.
    (e) Atropine is not effective for spinal block-induced nausea.

14. Factors affecting spinal blockade:
    (a) Baricity of local anaesthetic solution.
    (b) Site of injection.
    (c) Age.
    (d) Positioning of the patient.
    (e) Speed of injection of anaesthetic solution.

15. Needles used in spinal anaesthesia:
    (a) Pencil-point needles have an opening at the tip.
    (b) Both Quincke and Pitkin's needles have nerve-cutting edges.
    (c) Continuous spinal catheter can be introduced through Tuohy needle.
    (d) Cutting-edge needles give better tactile sensation of the layers of ligaments.
    (e) Greene needle has a non-cutting bevel.

16. Taylor approach:
    (a) Paramedian approach is directed towards L5–S1 interface.
    (b) Posterior superior iliac spine is one of the landmarks.
    (c) Significant resistance is seen with interspinous ligament.
    (d) Is best used in patients with difficulty in bending spine.
    (e) The needle is advanced in a cranio-caudal direction and at an angle of 55°.

17. Complications of spinal anaesthesia:
    (a) Paraesthesia is a risk factor for persistent neurological injury.
    (b) Multiple single-injection spinal anaesthesia can increase the risk of cauda equina.
    (c) Cauda equina syndrome can be prevented by aspirating CSF before and after the local anaesthetic injection.
    (d) Sterile water if injected can cause arachnoiditis.
    (e) Female gender is more prone to spinal haematoma.

18. Total spinal anaesthesia:
    (a) Most frequent cause is inadvertent spinal after epidural anaesthesia.
    (b) Hypertension is seen.
    (c) Usually resolves on its own.
    (d) Vasopressors may be required.
    (e) Tracheal intubation may be required.

19. Subdural block:
    (a) Mostly seen with epidural anaesthesia.
    (b) Subdural space is continuous with the cranial cavity.
    (c) Fast onset sensory block is seen.

(d) Trigeminal nerve palsy is seen.

(e) Respiratory complications may be seen.

20. Spinal haematoma;

(a) May occur in the absence of anticoagulant treatment.

(b) Increased age and history of bleeding increases the risk of spinal haematoma.

(c) Most spinal haematomas occur because of prominent epidural venous plexus.

(d) Conservative management is the best option.

21. Meningitis seen with spinal anaesthesia:

(a) Oral flora from practitioner not wearing mask can cause it.

(b) Aseptic type is always seen.

(c) The risk is increased with underlying collagen vascular disease.

(d) Most common organism causing is *Staphylococcus aureus*.

(e) Preservative-containing solutions can increase the risk.

22. Post-dural puncture headache;

(a) Incidence is low.

(b) Pain is felt due to increase in cerebral blood flow.

(c) Diplopia and tinnitus can be seen.

(d) May resolve spontaneously in 24 h.

(e) Blood patch is 100 % effective.

23. Post-dural puncture headache:

(a) Mostly seen in the temporal region.

(b) All cranial nerves can be affected.

(c) Patient may complain of double vision.

(d) Majority of patients see improvement within 24 h.

(e) Most of the headaches will require invasive treatment.

24. Post-dural puncture headache:
    (a) Bed rest is compulsory.
    (b) Caffeine reduces cerebral blood flow.
    (c) History of hypertonus is a contraindication to
        caffeine therapy.
    (d) Blood patches can be performed in
        immunosuppressed patients.
    (e) Sumatriptan can be used in place of caffeine.

25. Cardiovascular complications with spinal anaesthesia:
    (a) Excessive sedation can cause cardiac arrest.
    (b) Both left atrium and right atrium may contribute to
        the bradycardia.
    (c) Bradycardia should be aggressively treated.
    (d) Coronary perfusion pressure is central to CPR
        secondary to cardiac arrest seen with spinal
        anaesthesia.
    (e) Bradycardia responds to atropine.

26. Blood patch:
    (a) Forms a clot over the meningeal hole.
    (b) Symptoms resolve in 2–3 days after the block.
    (c) If first patch fails, second patch is not advised.
    (d) Most common complication of blood patch is
        backache.
    (e) Both caffeine and sumatriptan intravenously can
        treat PDPH.

27. Transient neurologic symptoms:
    (a) Mostly seen with spinal anaesthesia.
    (b) Motor symptoms may be seen.
    (c) More seen with hyperbaric lidocaine.
    (d) The most effective treatment is symptomatic.
    (e) Avoiding vasopressors to local anaesthetics may
        help prevent TNS.

28. Epidural block:
    (a) Aspirin use is a contraindication.
    (b) Can be placed 1 h after subcutaneous heparin.
    (c) INR <1.5 is sufficient for epidural placement.
    (d) Gp IIa/IIIb inhibitors should be stopped for 4 weeks before epidural placement.
    (e) Clopidogrel should be stopped for 24 h.

29. Epidural block anatomy:
    (a) Spinous processes angulate sharply in the cervical region.
    (b) Ligamentum flavum is made up of elastin fibres.
    (c) Destruction of at least three consecutive spinal nerve roots is required to produce a total sensory loss of the dermatome.
    (d) T4 is at the root of scapula.
    (e) Epidural space extends from the base of the skull to the sacral hiatus.

30. Epidural space:
    (a) Is a potential space.
    (b) Bounded laterally by pedicles and intervertebral foramen.
    (c) There is free fluid in the space.
    (d) Contains batson's venous plexus.
    (e) Is decreased in pregnancy.

31. Epidural injection:
    (a) Interspaces can be used in children from 4 years onwards.
    (b) Distance from skin to surface is 4–6 cm.
    (c) Proprioceptive fibres are blocked first.
    (d) Sympathetic block is always higher than sensory block.
    (e) High thoracic block show more dense sympathetic blocks.

32. Cardiovascular effects:
    (a) Dependent on blockade above T4 or below T4.
    (b) Stroke volume is decreased with neuraxial blockade.
    (c) A compensatory mechanism for decreased mean arterial pressure is vasoconstriction.
    (d) Decrease in blood pressure is more tolerated better in elderly than young.
    (e) Splanchnic nerve block with decrease in medullary secretion of catecholamines is seen.

33. Epidural anaesthesia:
    (a) Gastrointestinal visceral perfusion is preserved.
    (b) Urinary retention is seen.
    (c) Has a cardioprotective effect in those having atherosclerotic disease.
    (d) May provoke nausea.
    (e) Respiratory arrest may occur.

34. Epidural needle:
    (a) Tuohy needle can be 16 G or 18 G.
    (b) The curve at the tip is 15–30°.
    (c) Multiple hole catheters can be better than single hole.
    (d) Solution used for cleaning can cause arachnoiditis.
    (e) Midline sitting position is better in obese patients.

35. Techniques for space location:
    (a) Air has been found less reliable than a combination of air and lignocaine.
    (b) Use of air can give a patchy block.
    (c) Catheter should not be inserted >5 cm.
    (d) Excess use of saline may be avoided.
    (e) Air used for space localisation is better in children.

36. Complications of neuraxial block:
    (a) Epidural abscess requires immediate treatment.
    (b) Epidural hematoma may present as initial loss of consciousness.

(c) Catheter shearing warrants removal of catheter while the needle is still inside.

(d) The probability of developing post-dural puncture headache is very high.

(e) Urinary retention is seen with epidural catheters.

37. Sacrum:
    (a) Formed by fusion of fifth lumbar and four sacral vertebrae.
    (b) Sacral hiatus is due to failure of fifth pair of laminae.
    (c) Sacrococcygeal ligament is an extension of ligamentum flavum.
    (d) Sacral canal contains epidural venous plexus which terminates at S2.
    (e) Adipose tissue may be responsible for unpredictable segmental spread.

38. Caudal block:
    (a) Lateral position is more efficacious in children.
    (b) Posterior superior iliac spine forms base of triangle as one of the landmarks.
    (c) Fluoroscopy gives better visualisation of the spine.
    (d) A give-in feeling indicates entry into the space.
    (e) Dural sac extends lower in adults than in children.

39. Caudal block:
    (a) Clear CSF is not an indication for abandoning the procedure.
    (b) False give in can be seen with penetration of cancellous bone.
    (c) Subperiosteal injection is painful.
    (d) Electrical stimulation can be used to ascertain needle placement in children.
    (e) If injected within bone, it can cause toxicity.

40. Caudal block:
    (a) Causes autonomic and sensory block only.
    (b) Parasympathetic block leads to loss of bladder and intestine function.
    (c) Caudal space can accommodate large volumes of local anaesthetic.
    (d) Sacral canal only contains cauda equina.
    (e) Can be used for both upper and lower lumbar root surgery.

41. Caudal block:
    (a) Increase in dose is required in pregnant females.
    (b) Horner's syndrome can be seen in pregnant females.
    (c) Spread of block is more predictable in adults.
    (d) Can decrease the response to stress in children.
    (e) Percutaneous epidural neuroplasty is done for chronic low back pain.

42. Caudal block (complications):
    (a) Seizures are seen more with lumbar than thoracic epidurals.
    (b) The earliest changes seen on intravenous injection of local anaesthetic on ECG is an increase in QRS wave.
    (c) Total spinal anaesthesia can be seen in children.
    (d) Discitis and vertebral osteomyelitis is seen.
    (e) Higher levels of blockade can be achieved in children than adults.

43. Combined spinal epidural:
    (a) Widely used in obstetric practice.
    (b) Effective, rapid onset analgesia with minimum risk of toxicity or motor block.
    (c) Can cause significant reduction in the duration of the first stage of labour in primiparous parturients.

(d) Is superior to epidural for hip knee arthroplasty.
(e) Epidural volume extension allows faster motor recovery of lower limbs.

44. Combined spinal epidural block:
    (a) Posterior epidural space distance is important for needle-through-needle technique.
    (b) Skin to epidural space distance is mostly 8 cm.
    (c) Width of posterior epidural space is a constant throughout.
    (d) Ligamentum flavum can be always relied upon to give feel of entering epidural space.
    (e) Separate-needle technique is better than needle through needle.

45. Subarachnoid block:
    (a) Catheter migration into subarachnoid space is seen more with needle-through-needle technique than separate-needle technique.
    (b) CSE produces greater sensorimotor anaesthesia and prolonged recovery than single-shot spinal.
    (c) Neurological complications are seen more with needle-through-needle technique than single-shot spinal.
    (d) Needle-through-needle technique predisposes to metal toxicity.
    (e) Administration of intrathecal opioids decreases the incidence of post-dural puncture headache.

46. Combined spinal epidural:
    (a) Increased fetal bradycardia is seen with combined spinal epidural.
    (b) More complications seen with CSE done in sitting than lateral position.
    (c) PDPH is rarer if atraumatic needles are used.
    (d) Risk of infection and haematoma increases with multiples attempts.

Answers

1. (a) T   (b) F   (c) T   (d) F   (e) T

There are three curves—two anterior (cervical, lumbar) and one posterior (thoracic). Supraspinous ligament is ligamentum nuchae above C7. Ligamentum nuchae is seen in normal spine and connects laminae. Arachnoid mater ends at S2. There are five ligaments in spine. Supraspinous ligament connects apices of spinous processes. Interspinous ligament connects spinous processes. Ligamentum flavum connects laminae above and below. Anterior and posterior ligaments also connect the vertebrae. Filum terminale holds spinal cord to sacrum.

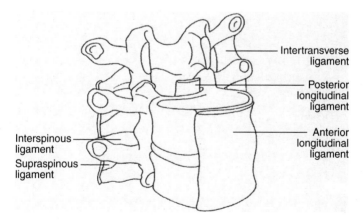

Fig: Ligaments of the vertebral column

2. (a) T   (b) F   (c) T   (d) F   (e) F

The structures traversed in median approach are skin, subcutaneous fat, supraspinous ligament, interspinous ligament, ligamentum flavum, dura mater, subdural space, arachnoid mater and subarachnoid space. The structures traversed in paramedian approach are skin, subcutaneous fat, ligamentum flavum, dura mater, subdural space, arachnoid mater and subarachnoid space. Spinal cord ends at L3 at birth and at L1 in adults. Iliac crest marks L4–L5 and is known as Tuffier's line. Umbilicus corresponds to T10. Cervical roots lie a space below their level of exit.

3. (a) F   (b) T   (c) F   (d) T   (e) F

   Dermatome is an area of skin innervated by sensory fibres from a single spinal nerve. The factors affecting local anaesthetics uptake are lipid content of the nervous tissue, concentration of local anaesthetic in CSF, surface area of nerve tissue exposed and blood flow to nerve tissue. Spaces of Virchow-Robin are areas of pia mater that surround blood vessels that penetrate central nervous system. They connect with perineural clefts that surround nerve cell bodies in spinal cord.

4. (a) F   (b) T   (c) T   (d) F   (e) T

   Spinal cord is supplied by numerous radicular arteries which form anterior spinal artery and twin posterior spinal arteries. Thoracolumbar segment of spinal cord (T8 to medullary cone) draws its arterial supply from large-calibre arteria radicularis magnus, which arises from an intercostals artery on left side. Cauda equina is supplied by branches of lumbar, iliolumbar, lateral or median sacral arteries. Posterior spinal artery arises from fourth segment of the vertebral artery and supply posterior one third of the spinal cord. The plexus is in anterolateral area of epidural space. They drain not only the spinal cord and its canal but also part of cerebrospinal fluid.

5. (a) T   (b) T   (c) F   (d) T   (e) T

6. (a) F   (b) F   (c) F   (d) T   (e) F

   Cerebrospinal fluid is produced at 0.35 ml/h. It is formed by active secretion and diffusion through the epithelial cells of choroid plexus, but also to a small extent in subarachnoid space and perivascularly. Obesity and pregnancy decreases cerebrospinal due to compression of intervertebral foramen and displacement of CSF. The approximate volume is 150 ml.

7. (a) T   (b) T   (c) F   (d) T

   Clonidine is an $\alpha 2$ agonist. It facilitates action of local anaesthetic without causing motor weakness when injected intrathecally. Neostigmine inhibits breakdown of acetylcholine and produces analgesia when injected intrathecally.

8. (a) F   (b) T   (c) T   (d) T   (e) T

   Renal blood flow is autoregulated above mean arterial blood pressure of 50 mmHg. The risk factors for hypotension are chronic alcohol consumption, history of hypertension, increased body mass index and increased sensory block height.

9. (a) F   (b) T   (c) F   (d) F   (e) F

   The unilateral block is intended to block anterior and posterior roots on the side of operation. Sympathetic fibres remain unblocked on contralateral side leading to low incidence of hypotension. There is a reduction in the extent of sympathetic block by 70 %. The recovery from anaesthesia is faster. Strict unilateral analgesia is rarely achieved.

10. (a) F   (b) T   (c) T   (d) T   (e) T

    Lateral decubitus position is used though occasionally paramedian is used which offers the best angle for catheter placement. The cause of transient neurological symptoms is sacral pooling of injected local anaesthetic due to the higher injection resistance in the microcatheter. A catheter should be removed with extreme caution. The patient is placed in the lateral position with the back flexed so as to stretch ligamentum flavum. Microcatheters cause an inflammatory reaction in area of puncture allowing sealing of the dural perforation site and thus prevent cerebrospinal loss.

11. (a) F   (b) T   (c) F   (d) T   (e) T

Preloading has not shown to be effective in preventing hypotension. The angle should not be more than 20° as greater angle will decrease cerebral perfusion and blood flow due to increase in JVP.

12. (a) T   (b) F   (c) F   (d) T

13. (a) T   (b) F   (c) F   (d) T   (e) F

Spinal anaesthesia does not normally affect lung parameters unless there is high spinal when expiratory reserve volume, peak expiratory flow rate and maximum minute ventilation decrease. Dyspnoea seen is usually due to inability to feel the chest wall move during respiration. Main muscles affected during high spinal anaesthesia are muscles of expiration. Increased peristalsis leads to nausea.

14. (a) T   (b) T   (c) T   (d) T   (e) T

Isobaric bupivacaine appears to increase block height whereas hyperbaric bupivacaine does not appear to change block height. Positioning of patient does not affect isobaric solutions.

15. (a) F   (b) T   (c) T   (d) F   (e) T

Sprotte and Whitacre needles are pencil-point needles with opening 2–4 mm proximal to the tip. Pencil-point needles give better tactile sensation.

16. (a) T   (b) F   (c) F   (d) T   (e) T

    The landmark is 1 cm medial and inferior to posterior superior iliac spine. The significant resistance is due to ligamentum flavum.

17. (a) T   (b) T   (c) T   (d) T   (e) T

    The causes of arachnoiditis are infection, myelogram from oil-based dyes, intrathecal blood and intrathecal steroids and trauma.

18. (a) T   (b) F   (c) F   (d) T   (e) T

    Clinical features are restlessness, breathing difficulties, hypotension and loss of consciousness. Total spinal can be life threatening and requires immediate treatment.

19. (a) F   (b) T   (c) F   (d) T   (e) T

    Subdural block is more associated with spinal anaesthesia or myelography. The subdural space is widest in cervical region and is continuous with the cranial cavity unlike epidural space. An unusually high sensory block is seen which develops slowly over a period of 20 min. Trigeminal nerve palsy and Horner's syndrome are seen. Respiratory complications are seen if the block is above T8 and are seen due to accompanying paralysis of the intercostals muscles.

20. (a) T   (b) T   (c) T   (d) F

    The risk factors for spinal haematoma are increased age, GIT bleeding, anticoagulant therapy, female gender and aspirin. Spinal haematoma is a surgical emergency.

21. (a) T   (b) F   (c) T   (d) T   (e) T

22. (a) F   (b) T   (c) T   (d) F   (e) F

    Incidence is 0.2–25 %. Pain is due to increased blood flow due to decreased cerebrospinal fluid to maintain volume. It takes 1–6 weeks for it to resolve spontaneously. Blood patch is effective in 64 % of PDPH due to obstetric causes and 95 % in non-obstetric causes.

23. (a) F   (b) F   (c) T   (d) F   (e) F

The headache is mainly occipito-frontal. All cranial nerves can be affected except olfactory nerve, glossopharyngeal nerve and vagus nerve. The most commonly affected nerves are abducens nerve and vestibulocochlear nerve. Abducens nerve may be involved with double vision, with parallel horizontal images and difficulties in focussing on objects. Most of the patients see complete recovery in 5–7 days. In 80 % of patients, the symptoms resolve within 2 weeks. More than 85 % patients get better with conservative measurement.

24. (a) T   (b) T   (c) T   (d) F   (e) T

Caffeine leads to cerebral vasoconstriction and decreased cerebral blood flow. Other contraindications to caffeine are history of epilepsy and pre-eclampsia. Blood patch is not done in immune suppressed because of risk of infection. Sumatriptan is a serotonin-type 1d receptor agonist.

25. (a) F   (b) T   (c) T   (d) T   (e) T

Excessive sedation can decrease preload and can cause respiratory depression leading to cardiac arrest. Low pressure baroreceptors in right atrium, receptors in myocardial pacemaker and mechanoreceptors in right atrium contribute to bradycardia. Successful CPR requires coronary perfusion pressure gradient between 15 and 20 mmHg.

26. (a) T   (b) F   (c) F   (d) T   (e) F

Symptoms usually resolve within 1–24 h after the block. Second patch has a success rate of 90 %. Most common complication after blood patch is backache, seen in 35 % of patients. Other complications seen are pain in the nape of neck, increased temperature and dizziness. Sumatriptan is given subcutaneously.

27. (a) T   (b) F   (c) T   (d) T   (e) T

Transient neurological symptoms are rarely seen after epidural. There are no neurological findings (motor, sensory or sphincter disturbances). The incidence is more with hyperbaric lidocaine, mepivacaine and intrathecal pethidine.

28. (a) F   (b) F   (c) T   (d) T   (e) F

Epidural can be placed 4 h after subcutaneous heparin and 12 h after low molecular weight heparin administration. Clopidogrel needs to be stopped for 7 days and ticlodipine for 4 days.

29. (a) F   (b) T   (c) T   (d) T   (e) T

Spinous processes have sharp angulation in mid-thoracic region with maximum angulation seen between T3–T7. The spinous processes in cervical, lower thoracic and lumbar region are horizontal.

30. (a) T   (b) T   (c) F   (d) T   (e) T

Batson's plexus is continuous with iliac vessels in pelvis and azygous system in abdominal and thoracic body walls. Epidural space is decreased in pregnancy because of engorgement of veins.

31. (a) F   (b) T   (c) F   (d) T   (e) T

Interspaces can be felt from 8 years onwards. The sequence of blockade is sympathetic fibres, pain fibres, temperature fibres, proprioceptive fibres and motor blockade. Sympathetic blockade is 0–4 segments higher than sensory blockade.

32. (a) T   (b) T   (c) T   (d) F   (e) T

Central venous pressure is increased with increase in stroke volume.

33. (a) T   (b) F   (c) T   (d) T   (e) T

Epidural anaesthesia has a cardioprotective effect in those having atherosclerotic disease. There is increased plasma norepinephrine after surgery which increases the nitric oxide causing vasospasm in endothelium of atherosclerotic disease. Sympathetic block causes decreased cardiac output and thus decreasing the blood flow causing brainstem ischaemia.

34. (a) T   (b) T   (c) T   (d) T   (e) T

35. (a) T   (b) T   (c) T   (d) T   (e) F

Excess use of saline dilutes the local anaesthetic causing inadequate block.

36. (a) T   (b) T   (c) F   (d) T   (e) T

Main cause of epidural abscess is *Staphylococcus aureus.* The symptoms are high fever, cervicothoracic/lumbar pain. Immediate surgical treatment within 12 h is required. Epidural hematoma may present with loss of consciousness, severe pain, neurological disturbance, Cheyne stokes respiration and bradycardia. The catheter and the needle are always removed simultaneously if catheter is stuck. Force should never be used while pulling. If required, wait for the patient to stand up and pull catheter during flexion or slight extension of back. There is a 70–80 % chance of post-dural puncture headache.

37. (a) F   (b) T   (c) T   (d) F   (e) T

Sacrum is formed by fusion five sacral vertebrae. Sacral venous plexus terminates at S4.

38. (a) T   (b) T   (c) T   (d) T   (e) F

Lateral position is more efficacious in children and prone position in adults. A give-in feeling indicates entry into sacrococcygeal ligament. Dural sac extends lower in children than adults.

39. (a) F   (b) T   (c) T   (d) T   (e) T

The procedure should be abandoned on visualisation of CSF and blood. The cortical layer of sacral bone is thin especially in infants and older subjects and can give a false in feeling. Electrical stimulation can be used for needle placement. S2–S4 contraction can be seen with 1–10 mA. If local anaesthetic is injected in bone marrow, toxicity can occur because of rapid absorption.

40. (a) F   (b) T   (c) T   (d) F   (e) F

Caudal block causes autonomic, sensory and motor block. Caudal block leads to loss of visceromotor function of bladder and intestine distal to colonic splenic flexure. Caudal space can accommodate 10–25 ml of local anaesthetic. Sacral canal contains spinal meninges, adipose tissue and sacral venous plexus in addition to cauda equina.

41. (a) F   (b) T   (c) F   (d) T   (e) T

The dose requirement is decreased in pregnant females because of congestion of veins. Horner's syndrome can be seen with larger doses and with patient positioned supine. Spread of block is more predictable up to 12 years of age.

42. (a) T   (b) F   (c) T   (d) T   (e) T

The earliest changes seen are T wave changes.

43. (a) T   (b) T   (c) T   (d) T   (e) T

44. (a) T   (b) F   (c) F   (d) F   (e) T

Underestimation of posterior epidural space can lead to higher block failure. Skin to epidural space distance is between 4 and 6 cm in 80 % of patients. Width of posterior epidural space is widest in mid-lumbar and decreases towards cervical vertebral column. There may be gaps in ligamentum flavum which cannot be relied upon. Separate-needle technique is better than needle-through-needle technique because catheter is separately placed prior to initiation of block, thereby decreasing the risk of neurologic injury.

45. (a) T   (b) T   (c) T   (d) F   (e) T

Neurological complications are seen with 37 % of patients in needle-through-needle technique as compared to 9 % in single-shot spinal technique.

46. (a) T   (b) T   (c) T   (d) T

9 Regional Anaesthesia in Obstetrics

1. Anatomic changes seen in pregnancy:
   (a) Decreased CSF volume.
   (b) Increased sensory blockade.
   (c) Epidural and vertebral veins are enlarged.
   (d) Lumbar lordosis and thoracic kyphosis is altered.
   (e) Interspinous spaces are narrowed.

2. Physiologic changes seen in pregnancy:
   (a) Are due to hormones secreted by corpus luteum and placenta.
   (b) Oxygen consumption is decreased.
   (c) Lower arterial pressure is seen.
   (d) Oestrogen leads to decreased vascular resistance.
   (e) Blood volume is increased.

3. Cardiovascular changes seen in pregnancy:
   (a) Increase in heart rate and decrease in cardiac output is seen.
   (b) Decrease in peripheral vascular resistance is seen.
   (c) Lower arterial pressure is seen.
   (d) Left axis deviation may be normal.
   (e) Premature atrial contractions may be seen.

4. Respiratory changes seen in pregnancy:
   (a) Minute ventilation decreases.
   (b) Dead space is increased.
   (c) Alveolar ventilation is increased.
   (d) Elevation of diaphragm is normally seen.
   (e) There are no changes in lung volumes.

R. Gupta, D. Patel, *Multiple Choice Questions in Regional Anaesthesia*,
DOI 10.1007/978-3-642-31257-1_9, © Springer-Verlag Berlin Heidelberg 2013

5. Respiratory changes seen in pregnancy:
    (a) Total lung capacity remains unchanged.
    (b) Functional residual capacity is always
        asymptomatic.
    (c) Residual volume never comes back to pre-pregnancy
        levels.
    (d) Women are more prone to mucous membrane bleeds.
    (e) Trendelberg position contributes
        to hypoxia.

6. Metabolic changes seen in pregnancy:
    (a) Oxygen consumption increases by 20 % at term.
    (b) Partial pressures of both carbon dioxide and oxygen
        are decreased.
    (c) Uptake of inhalational anaesthetics is enhanced.
    (d) Increased metabolic rate may contribute to
        hypoxemia.
    (e) pH remains unchanged.

7. Gastrointestinal changes seen in pregnancy:
    (a) Decreased gastrointestinal motility is seen.
    (b) Lower oesophageal tone is increased by first
        trimester.
    (c) Gastric emptying is progressively delayed.
    (d) Metoclopramide hastens gastric emptying.
    (e) Transient neurologic symptoms may be seen with
        dopamine antagonists.

8. Endocrine changes seen in pregnancy:
    (a) Plasma volume increases at term.
    (b) Sodium retention is seen.
    (c) Serum cholinesterase activity is decreased
        by 50 % below normal.
    (d) Albumin concentration decreases.
    (e) Hyperglycaemia and ketosis may be seen even in non
        diabetics.

9. Drug responses in pregnancy:
   (a) Neural sensitivity to local anaesthetics is increased.
   (b) Increased spread of local anaesthetic is seen when given neuraxially.
   (c) Minimum alveolar concentration for inhalational agents is decreased.
   (d) Progesterone increases the MAC for inhalational anaesthetics.
   (e) Lower doses of local anaesthetic are needed per dermatomal segment.

10. Placental transfer of drugs:
    (a) The drugs pass by active movement.
    (b) Placental transfer is modified by maternal drug concentrations.
    (c) Non-ionised drug is more lipophilic.
    (d) Acidosis increases the risk of ion trapping.
    (e) Local anaesthetics are weak acids.

11. Drug toxicity:
    (a) Fetus can excrete local anaesthetics back into maternal circulation.
    (b) 2-Chlorprocaine is the most toxic local anaesthetic for fetus.
    (c) Half-life of lidocaine is longer in newborns.
    (d) Bupivacaine can cause neonatal jaundice.
    (e) Neurologic changes may be seen with regional anaesthesia in newborns.

12. Uteroplacental blood flow:
    (a) Is autoregulated.
    (b) Pain may decrease the flow.
    (c) Neuraxial anaesthesia may decrease the flow.
    (d) Epinephrine containing local anaesthetics has no effect on the flow.
    (e) Test dose given in epidural does not effect the flow.

13. Pain in labour:
     (a) Pain in first stage is due to both cervix and uterus.
     (b) Upper thoracic dermatomes are affected in early labour.
     (c) Second-stage pain is mediated by pudendal nerve.
     (d) Epidural analgesia decreases maternal catecholamine secretions.
     (e) Maternal pain can cause reduce fetal arterial oxygen tension.

14. Pain in labour:
     (a) Has both visceral and somatic components.
     (b) Early labour pain is somatic.
     (c) Afferent nerves pass through paracervical plexus.
     (d) Pain may be referred to abdominal muscles and back.
     (e) Somatic pain is transferred by pudendal nerve.

15. Opioids for labour analgesia:
     (a) Meperidine is safe.
     (b) Meperidine has a short half-life in neonates.
     (c) Remifentanil has a short half-life.
     (d) Butorphanol has a ceiling effect on depression of ventilation.
     (e) Naloxone should be given to mother immediately before delivery.

16. Epidural analgesia in parturient:
     (a) Fetal monitoring is easy in lateral position.
     (b) Cardiac output is decreased in lateral position.
     (c) Sitting position is advantageous in obese women.
     (d) Epidural spread is more seen in supine patient.
     (e) Complications are less with midline approach.

17. Epidural analgesia in labour:
     (a) T10–L1 needs to be blocked for first stage.

(b) Second stage needs blockade of S2–S4.
(c) Epidural analgesia may prolong first stage of labour.
(d) Epidural analgesia may prolong second stage of labour.
(e) Prolonged second stage is more than 2 h in multiparous and 3 h in nulliparous.

18. Patient-controlled epidural analgesia:
    (a) Has good maternal acceptance.
    (b) A demand bolus dose of 4 ml with a lockout period of 10 min gives best results.
    (c) Caudal approach is preferable.
    (d) Caudal analgesia has higher complication rate.
    (e) Rectal examination should be done before caudal injection.

19. Epidural catheters:
    (a) Multiple orifice catheters are better than single orifice.
    (b) Flexible tip catheters have high incidence of paraesthesias.
    (c) Short length of catheter insertion is more successful.
    (d) Catheter may migrate out as the patient changes position.
    (e) Optimal length of catheter insertion is 4–6 cm.

20. Paracervical block:
    (a) Is effective for first stage of labour.
    (b) Higher incidence of fetal asphyxia.
    (c) Involves submucosal injection near vaginal fornix.
    (d) Poor neonatal outcome has been seen with the use of bupivacaine.
    (e) Uterine curettage can be comfortably performed.

21. Test dose for epidural:
    (a) Is used to rule out inadvertent intravascular or intrathecal catheter placement.

(b) A small dose of local anaesthetic is used.
(c) Epinephrine increases sensitivity of the test dose.
(d) Epinephrine may decrease uteroplacental perfusion.
(e) Electrocardiography, peak to peak heart rate variation, may improve intrathecal detection.

22. Epinephrine as a test dose:
(a) Parturients have attenuated chronotropic response to vasopressors.
(b) Epinephrine efficacy is increased if injected during uterine diastole.
(c) Has no effect on uteroplacental perfusion.
(d) May cause fetal distress.
(e) May be dangerous in pre-eclampsia.

23. Combined spinal epidural for labour:
(a) Onset of analgesia is rapid.
(b) Can be used to cause analgesia without sympathectomy.
(c) Has been shown to decrease the number of instrumental deliveries.
(d) Incidence of dural puncture is decreased as compared to epidural analgesia.
(e) May cause more rapid cervical dilation.

24. Complications of combined spinal epidural in obstetrics:
(a) Fetal bradycardia is more seen.
(b) An increase incidence of emergency caesarean sections is seen.
(c) Increased incidence of post-dural puncture headache is seen.
(d) Increased intrathecal toxicity of medications may be seen.
(e) Aphasia or dysphagia may be seen.

25. Local anaesthetics for labour analgesia:
(a) 2-Chloprocaine is ideal local anaesthetic.

   (b) Sodium bisulphite can cause neurologic deficit.
   (c) EDTA is a safe substitute for sodium bisulphite.
   (d) Lipid-encapsulated preparations can provide pain relief for 48 h.
   (e) Delayed respiratory depression is seen with opioids.

26. Aortocaval compression syndrome:
   (a) Is due to pressure of uterus on inferior vena cava.
   (b) Fetal hypoxia may be seen.
   (c) There is no collateral circulation.
   (d) Volume loading is effective in preventing the syndrome.
   (e) Ephedrine is the vasopressor of choice.

27. Paracervical block in pregnancy:
   (a) Is useful for second stage of labour.
   (b) Does not prevent pain due to perineal stretch.
   (c) Both fornices are injected.
   (d) Post-partum neuropathy is a known complication.
   (e) Most common fetal complication is bradycardia.

28. Pudendal nerve block in obstetrics:
   (a) Pudendal nerve supplies only sensory innervations to vagina and perineum.
   (b) Is effective in second stage of labour.
   (c) Has a high success rate.
   (d) Early pudendal nerve block increases incidence of instrumental delivery.
   (e) Retroperitoneal haematomas is a known complication.

29. Hypertensive disorder in pregnancy:
   (a) Are seen in majority of the patients.
   (b) Blood pressure consistently above 5 % is a diagnostic criterion.
   (c) Seen more in nulliparous women.
   (d) Presence of oedema is must for diagnosis.
   (e) Placental ischaemia is the incriminating factor.

30. Hypertensive disorders manifest as:
    (a) Disseminated intravascular coagulation.
    (b) Oedema.
    (c) Proteinuria.
    (d) Decreased production of prostaglandin E.
    (e) Endothelial cell injury.

31. Severe pre-eclampsia is associated with:
    (a) Systolic blood pressure >15 % above baseline.
    (b) Proteinuria of 1 g/24 h.
    (c) Anuria.
    (d) Epigastric pain.
    (e) Visual disturbances.

32. Clinical manifestation seen with severe pre-eclampsia/ eclampsia:
    (a) Cortical blindness.
    (b) Hyporeflexia.
    (c) Cerebral haemorrhage.
    (d) Heart failure.
    (e) Liver necrosis.

33. Renal findings in severe eclampsia/pre-eclampsia:
    (a) Swelling of glomerular endothelial cells.
    (b) Reduced clearance of urea and creatinine.
    (c) Mean plasma volume is increased.
    (d) Renal blood flow is decreased.
    (e) Exaggerated retention of water and sodium is seen.

34. HELLP syndrome:
    (a) Consumption coagulopathy is seen.
    (b) Paradoxical thrombocytosis is seen.
    (c) Bleeding time is a reliable indicator of clotting.
    (d) Elevated liver enzymes can be seen.

(e) Prolongation of prothrombin and partial thromboplastin times indicate consumption coagulopathy.

35. Management of hypertensive disorder in pregnancy:
    (a) Correction of clotting abnormalities should be the aim.
    (b) Magnesium is used for convulsions.
    (c) Anti-hypertensive medications are not required.
    (d) Hydralazine is the preferred anti-hypertensive agent.
    (e) Delivery should be done in severe cases.

36. Regional anaesthesia in hypertensive disorders:
    (a) Clotting abnormalities is an absolute contraindication.
    (b) Volume-depleted patients may respond better to epidural anaesthesia.
    (c) Intervillous blood flow is increased with epidural anaesthesia.
    (d) Amide local anaesthetics may cause toxicity.
    (e) Higher doses of vasopressors are required to correct hypotension.

37. Antepartum haemorrhage:
    (a) Most common cause is placenta previa.
    (b) Maternal mortality is high with placenta previa.
    (c) Painless bleeding suggests placenta previa.
    (d) Placenta accreta is associated with less bleeding.
    (e) Bleeding may be concealed in abruption placenta.

38. Continuous spinal anaesthesia in obstetrics:
    (a) Faster onset of anaesthesia and analgesia.
    (b) Useful in high-risk patients.
    (c) Antacid administration is not required.
    (d) Spinal catheter can be used for 48 h.
    (e) Opioids injected intrathecally can cause hypotension.

39. Epidural anaesthesia:
    (a) Increased requirement of local anaesthetic dose is required.
    (b) Negative pressure is increased during pregnancy.
    (c) Cervix opening has no bearing on the epidural efficacy.
    (d) Lidocaine has higher umbilical blood levels after injection.
    (e) Left lateral displacement of uterus until birth of the child is required.

40. Complications of regional anaesthesia:
    (a) Incidence of pruritus is high with CSE as compared to the epidural.
    (b) Incidence of intraoperative shivering is decreased by epidural administration of opioids.
    (c) Epidural anaesthesia may cause fever.
    (d) Epidural blood patch has no side effects.
    (e) Most common nerve injury seen is to ulnar nerve.

Answers

1. (a) T (b) T (c) T (d) T (e) T

2. (a) T (b) F (c) T (d) T (e) T
   Oxygen consumption is increased during pregnancy.
   Decreased vascular resistance is due to oestrogen,
   progesterone and prostacyclin.

3. (a) T (b) T (c) T (d) T (e) T
   Increase in heart rate (15–20 %) and cardiac output (up to
   50 %) is seen. Lower vascular resistance is found in uterine,
   renal and other vascular beds. These changes result in a
   lower arterial pressure. Increase in cardiac output is seen
   due to added blood volume. Left axis deviation is caused
   by upward displacement of heart and gravid uterus.

4. (a) F (b) F (c) T (d) T (e) F
   Minute ventilation increases 50 % above normal by term.
   This comes back to normal within 3 weeks after delivery.
   This is due to 40 % increase in tidal volume and a small
   increase in respiratory rate. There is no change in dead
   space. Alveolar ventilation increases by 70 % at term.
   Expiratory reserve volume, residual volume and functional
   residual capacity decrease by third semester of pregnancy.

5. (a) T (b) F (c) F (d) T (e) T
   Decreased functional residual capacity is mostly
   asymptomatic, but those with pre-existing alterations in
   closing volume (smoking, obesity, scoliosis, pulmonary

disease) may expect early airway closure leading to hypoxaemia. Residual volume and functional residual capacity return back to normal shortly after delivery.

6. (a) T   (b) F   (c) T   (d) T   (e) T

Increased alveolar ventilation leads to decrease in partial pressure of carbon dioxide and increased partial pressure of oxygen. Maternal uptake and elimination of inhalational anaesthetics are enhanced because of increase alveolar ventilation and decreased functional residual capacity.

7. (a) T   (b) F   (c) T   (d) T   (e) T

Enlarged progesterone production causes decreased gastrointestinal motility and slower absorption of food. Gastric secretions are more acidic and lower oesophageal sphincter tone is decreased. Delay in gastric emptying can be demonstrated by the end of the first trimester. Uterine growth leads to upward displacement and rotation of stomach with increased pressure and further delay in gastric emptying. Dopamine antagonists hasten gastric emptying and increased lower oesophageal sphincter tone.

8. (a) T   (b) T   (c) F   (d) T   (e) T

Plasma volume and total blood volume increase by 40–50 % and 25–40 %, respectively, by term. Sodium retention and increased body water content is seen due to an increased mineralocorticoid activity. Plasma cholinesterase activity decreases by 20 % below normal. Albumin concentration decreases, and there is increase in free fraction of protein-bound drugs. Human placental lactogen and cortisol increase tendency to hyperglycaemia and ketosis.

9. (a) T   (b) T   (c) T   (d) F   (e) T

Neural sensitivity to local anaesthetic is increased because of progesterone. Increased spread of local anaesthetic is seen due to epidural venous engagement and enhanced sensitivity to local anaesthetic block. Minimum alveolar concentration for inhalational agents is decreased by 8–12 weeks of gestation.

10. (a) F   (b) T   (c) T   (d) T   (e) F

The drugs cross placenta by simple diffusion. Factors affecting placental transfer include physiochemical characteristics of drug, maternal drug concentrations and properties of placenta. With acidosis, there is greater tendency for the drug to exist in ionised form which cannot diffuse back across the placenta. This is called ion trapping.

11. (a) T   (b) F   (c) T   (d) T   (e) T

2-Chloprocaine is the only drug that is metabolised in fetal blood quickly that does not accumulate. Half-life of lidocaine is greater in newborns because of greater volume of distribution and tissue uptake. Bupivacaine can cause neonatal jaundice because of its high affinity for fetal erythrocyte membrane resulting in increased friability causing hemolysis. Neurologic and adaptive functional changes may be seen with regional anaesthesia which lasts for less than 48 h.

12. (a) F   (b) T   (c) T   (d) T   (e) T

Uteroplacental blood flow is not autoregulated and is dependent on maternal blood pressure. Pain causes hyperventilation which can decrease uteroplacental blood flow. Neuraxial blocks may cause uterine hypertonicity decreasing flow.

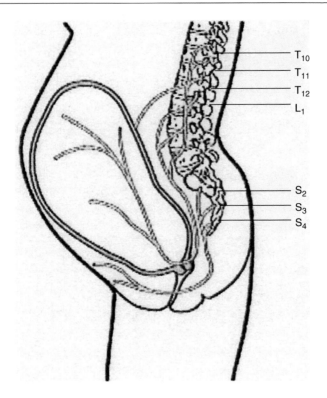

Nerves involved with labour at different stages

13. (a) T   (b) F   (c) T   (d) T   (e) T

First stage labour pain is caused by uterine contractions related to dilation of cervix and distension of lower uterine segment. Only lower thoracic dermatomes (T11–T12) are affected in early labour. During the second stage, impulse due to distension in vaginal vault and perineum are carried by pudendal nerve (S2–S4).

14.   (a) T   (b) F   (c) T   (d) T   (e) T

Visceral stimulation occurs due to involvement of cervix and lower uterine segment dilation. Early labour pain is primarily visceral and occurs during uterine contractions. Afferent impulses are transmitted via pudendal nerve through the sacral plexus to spinal cord at S234.

15.   (a) F   (b) F   (c) T   (d) T   (e) F

Meperidine leads to formation of normeperidine which can cause seizures. The drug can also cause nausea and vomiting, dose-related depression of ventilation, orthostatic hypotension, neonatal depression and euphoria. Meperidine may cause alterations of fetal heart rate, decreased beat to beat variability and tachycardia. Meperidine has a long half-life (62 h). Remifentanil is rapidly metabolised by serum and tissue cholinesterases and has a short (3 min) context sensitive half-life. Naloxone should not be administered to the mother shortly before delivery to prevent neonatal ventilator depression because it reverses neonatal depression.

16.   (a) T   (b) T   (c) T   (d) F   (e) F

Maternal position has no effect on epidural spread. Minor complications (difficulty in threading catheter, paraesthesias, venous cannulation) are seen with midline approach.

17.   (a) T   (b) T   (c) F   (d) T   (e) T

Early initiation of epidural analgesia during latent phase of labour (2–4 cm of dilation) may result in prolongation of first stage of labour and a higher incidence of dystocia. A prolongation of second stage is seen in nulliparous women due to decrease in expulsive forces or malpresentation of vertex.

18. (a) T   (b) T   (c) T   (d) T   (e) T

Caudal approach may result in faster onset of perineal analgesia. The complications involved are painful needle placement, increased failure rate, contamination of injection site and accident fetal injection. Rectal examination should be done to exclude needle placement in fetal-presenting part.

19. (a) T   (b) F   (c) T   (d) T   (e) T

There is less likelihood of patchy or unilateral block with multi-orifice catheters. Flexible tip catheters have lower incidence of catheter-induced paraesthesias and venous cannulations.

20. (a) T   (b) T   (c) T   (d) T   (e) T

There is association with fetal hypoxia and poor neonatal outcome. This may be related to uterine artery constriction or increased uterine tone.

21. (a) T   (b) T   (c) F   (d) T   (e) T

A small dose of local anaesthetic (lidocaine 45 mg or bupivacaine 5 mg) produces a readily identifiable sensory and motor block. Epinephrine test dose is controversial as it is associated with false positives.

22. (a) T   (b) T   (c) F   (d) T   (e) T

23. (a) T   (b) T   (c) T   (d) T   (e) T

Opioid only CSE analgesia can be used for analgesia without sympathectomy. It is especially useful in patients in whom a rapid decrease in intravascular volume is undesirable.

24. (a) T   (b) F   (c) T   (d) T   (e) T

An acute decrease in maternal epinephrine, seen after neuraxial analgesia, results in temporary imbalance of uterine tocolytic and urodynamic forces, resulting in uterine hypertonus and a decrease in uterine perfusion causing bradycardia. Drugs injected into the epidural space after CSE block may traverse the dural hole and result in increased CSF concentrations.

25. (a) T   (b) T   (c) F   (d) T   (e) T

2-Chlorprocaine provides rapid onset and reliable block with minimal risk of systemic toxicity. It is local anaesthetic of choice in presence of fetal acidosis. Increased neurotoxicity is seen with solutions containing sodium bisulphite at low pH. Severe spasmodic back pain has been described after large volume injection of solutions containing ethylenediaminetetraacetic acid. This is due to EDTA-induced binding of calcium from paravertebral muscles. Lipid-encapsulated morphine preparation can provide pain relief for 48 h after caesarean section.

26. (a) T   (b) T   (c) F   (d) T   (e) T

A collateral circulation occurs via the azygous vein system.

27. (a) F   (b) T   (c) T   (d) T   (e) T

Paracervical block provides adequate analgesia for first stage of labour before fetal descent. Five to ten millilitre of dilute local anaesthetic is injected by introducing needle through the vagina into left and right lateral vaginal fornix to a depth of 2–3 cm. Post-partum neuropathy may be seen due to direct sacral plexus trauma.

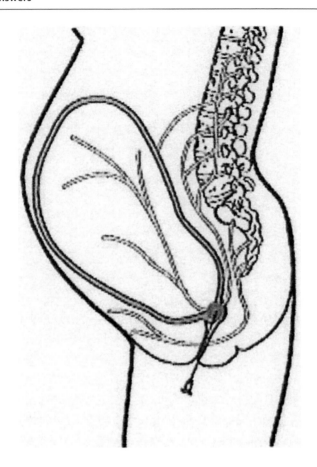

28. (a) F   (b) T   (c) F   (d) F   (e) T
Pudendal nerve also supplies vulva and provides motor innervations to perineal muscles and external anal sphincter. Success rate for bilateral pudendal nerve block is less than 50 %. Pudendal nerve block just before or after cervical dilation provides better analgesia and does not increase the incidence of instrumental delivery.

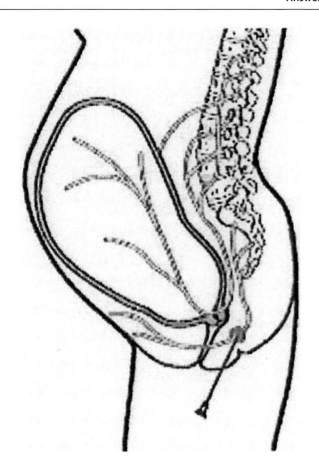

29. (a) F   (b) F   (c) T   (d) F   (e) T

Hypertensive disorders are seen in 7 % of patients with pregnancy. Blood pressure consistently above 15 % is diagnostic. It is predominantly seen in nulliparous young women. Presence of oedema is no longer necessary. Placental ischaemia results in secretion of renin which leads to vasoconstriction due to angiotensin.

30. (a) T   (b) T   (c) T   (d) T   (e) T

The platelets are fixed at the site of the endothelial damage resulting in abnormal coagulation causing disseminated intravascular coagulation. Increased angiotensin-mediated aldosterone secretion leads to release of thromboplastin with subsequent deposition of fibrin in glomerular vessels leading to proteinuria.

31. (a) T   (b) F   (c) F   (d) T   (e) T

A consistent systolic and diastolic pressure 15 % above baseline is seen. Proteinuria should be >5 g/24 h. Oliguria (400 ml/24 h) is seen.

32. (a) T   (b) F   (c) T   (d) T   (e) T

Hyperreflexia is seen. Cerebral haemorrhage and oedema are leading causes of death. Heart failure occurs because of peripheral vasoconstriction and hemoconcentration. Blood supply to liver is decreased leading to necrosis.

33. (a) T   (b) T   (c) F   (d) T   (e) T

The mean plasma volume in women with pre-eclampsia decreases by 9 %.

34. (a) T   (b) F   (c) F   (d) T   (e) T

Mild thrombocytopenia is seen. Bleeding time is prolonged in 25 % of patients with normal platelet counts and is not a reliable test of clotting.

35. (a) T   (b) T   (c) F   (d) T   (e) T

The management relies on prevention and control of convulsions, improving organ perfusion, controlling blood pressure and correct clotting. Magnesium is used to prevent convulsions. A loading dose of 4 g in 20 % solution is given over 5 min followed by an infusion of 1–2 g/h. Anti-hypertensives are used to lessen risk of cerebral haemorrhage. Hydralazine is preferred as it increases uteroplacental and renal blood flow.

36. (a) T (b) T (c) T (d) T (e) F

Volume-depleted patients positioned with left uterine displacement do not drop their blood pressure with use of epidural anaesthesia. Epidural anaesthesia is known to improve placental perfusion. Body clearance of amide local anaesthetics is prolonged in pre-eclampsia. There is an increased sensitivity to vasopressors in pre-eclampsia; therefore, lower doses are required.

37. (a) F (b) F (c) T (d) F (e) T

Abruption placenta occurs in 0.2–0.4 % of pregnancies, whereas placenta previa occurs in 0.1 % of pregnancies. Mortality seen with abruption placenta is 1.8–11 % as compared to 0.9 % in placenta previa. Placenta previa is associated with painless, bright-red vaginal bleeding usually after seventh month of pregnancy. Placenta accreta is penetration of myometrium by placental villi and risk of severe bleeding is increased.

38. (a) T (b) T (c) F (d) F (e) T

Spinal catheter should not be left >24 h because of increased incidence of post-dural puncture headache. Opioids can lead to slight decrease in blood pressure (<15 %).

39. (a) F (b) F (c) F (d) T (e) T

Epidural space narrows due to venous dilation and less dose is required. Insertion of an epidural catheter and administration of local anaesthetic is more effective when cervix is 5–6 cm open in primipara and 3–4 cm in nullipara. Concentrations of lidocaine and mepivacaine are higher as compared to ropivacaine, bupivacaine and etidocaine.

40. (a) T   (b) T   (c) T   (d) F   (e) F

Most cases of pruritus are self-limited and need no treatment. Epidural anaesthesia is associated with low-grade maternal fever. The most common complication of blood patch is backache. Most common nerves injured are lateral femoral cutaneous nerve and femoral nerve.

10 Regional Anaesthesia in Paediatrics

1. Regional anaesthesia in paediatrics:
   (a) Consent should not be obtained.
   (b) Mostly done after child is asleep.
   (c) Earliest parameter to change in toxicity is ECG.
   (d) Complications are less as compared to adults.
   (e) Dose required is more than adults.

2. Benefits of regional anaesthesia with general anaesthesia in paediatrics:
   (a) Pain relief.
   (b) Decreased use of anaesthetic agents.
   (c) Decreased incidence of nausea and vomiting.
   (d) Decreased risk of bleeding.
   (e) Malignant hyperthermia.

3. Contraindications of regional anaesthesia:
   (a) Infection at the site.
   (b) Degenerative axonal disease.
   (c) Coagulopathy.
   (d) Myelomeningocele.
   (e) Myopathies.

4. Respiratory considerations in infants:
   (a) Alveoli are mature at birth.
   (b) Diaphragm has more horizontal attachment.
   (c) Closing volume occurs within tidal volume.
   (d) Narrow airways contribute to resistance up to the age of 8 years.
   (e) Apnoea is seen more in preterm neonates.

R. Gupta, D. Patel, *Multiple Choice Questions in Regional Anaesthesia*,
DOI 10.1007/978-3-642-31257-1_10, © Springer-Verlag Berlin Heidelberg 2013

5. Cardiovascular considerations in infants:
   (a) Pulmonary vascular resistance falls at birth.
   (b) Cardiac output is less than the adults.
   (c) Atropine is the drug of choice for bradycardia.
   (d) Midline defects are associated with cardiac defects.
   (e) Autonomic function is fully functional at birth.

6. Thermoregulation in infants:
   (a) High-surface area to volume ratio leads to poor thermoregulation.
   (b) Brown fat is deficient in infants.
   (c) Radiation predominantly is responsible for heat loss in infants.
   (d) Neutral thermal environment for infants is at 28°.
   (e) Clotting factors are unaffected above temperatures of 28°.

7. Anatomical considerations for regional anaesthesia:
   (a) Tip of spinal cord is L3 at birth.
   (b) Meninges are at the same level as spinal cord at birth.
   (c) Fibrous strands are the hallmark of paediatric epidural space.
   (d) Myelination of nerves continues up to 3 years of age.
   (e) Resistance to epidural blockade of L5 to S1 is seen in infants.

8. Local anaesthetics:
   (a) Neonates have lesser capacity to oxidise and reduce amide local anaesthetic agents.
   (b) Conjugation of local anaesthetics reaches adult level by 3 months of age.
   (c) Clearance of drugs is similar in children.
   (d) Steady-state volume of distribution is increased as compared to adults.
   (e) Amino esters have rapid clearance in adults.

9. Toxicity of local anaesthetics:
   (a) Dose calculation in predicted volumes helps reduce toxicity.
   (b) An allergic reaction to esters is not seen.
   (c) Generalised convulsions are never seen.
   (d) May cause negative chronotropic effects.
   (e) Increased pulmonary vascular resistance is seen.

10. Bupivacaine in children:
    (a) Can be used as 0.1 % for continuous infusions.
    (b) Neonates and infants tolerate higher dose than older children.
    (c) The free fraction of bupivacaine may be greater causing more toxicity.
    (d) D-isomer is associated with most adverse effects.
    (e) Incidence of cardiotoxicity is more than neurotoxicity.

11. Ropivacaine in paediatrics:
    (a) Is an amide anaesthetic.
    (b) L enantiomer is more toxic.
    (c) Causes less of motor block.
    (d) Cardiovascular toxicity is seen.
    (e) Longer duration of action is seen as compared to mepivacaine.

12. Epidural analgesia:
    (a) Post-operative benefits are not seen.
    (b) Conus medullaris is lower as compared to adults in the epidural space.
    (c) Sacral vertebrae fuse by 8 years of age.
    (d) Catheter in caudal space is easier to insert.
    (e) There is increase chance of dura puncture during caudal injection.

13. Drugs in epidural anaesthesia:
    (a) Bupivacaine and ropivacaine are most commonly used.
    (b) Age is a better correlate than body weight for predicting spread.
    (c) 2-Chlorprocaine is better tolerated in neonates.
    (d) Ropivacaine has vasoconstricting action.
    (e) Ropivacaine should be used cautiously in patients with impaired hepatic function.

14. Adjuvants used in addition to local anaesthetic:
    (a) Epinephrine is used in a concentration of 1:200,000.
    (b) Opioids are more associated with adverse effects.
    (c) Clonidine acts on medullispinal pathways.
    (d) Psychomimetic side effects are not seen at low doses of ketamine (0.25–0.5 mg/kg)
    (e) Midazolam given epidurally acts as an analgesic agent.

15. Complications associated with epidural and caudal analgesia:
    (a) Epidural haematoma is extremely rare.
    (b) Sacral osteomyelitis is a known complication of caudal epidural.
    (c) Perforation of rectum can be avoided by introducing the needle steeply.
    (d) Blood patch is not effective in children.
    (e) Caffeine is not used in children for PDPH.

16. Local anaesthetic toxicity:
    (a) Heart rate is a sensitive marker for intravascular placement for epinephrine.
    (b) Incremental dosing reduces adverse effects.
    (c) Avoiding opioids helps reduce side effects.
    (d) Dilute solutions of local anaesthetics help avoid toxicity.
    (e) Sharp-tipped needles should be avoided.

17. Adverse effects of local anaesthetics:
     (a) Pruritus has the highest incidence.
     (b) Clonidine has higher incidence of itching than opioids.
     (c) Incidence of sedation is more in children as
         compared to adults.
     (d) Low-dose naloxone infusions help prevent itching,
         nausea and bowel complications.
     (e) Urinary retention may need catheterisation.

18. Epidural catheter insertion:
     (a) Negative aspiration of catheter has high sensitivity.
     (b) ECG has more specificity than negative aspiration.
     (c) Electrical stimulation can be used for catheter
         placement.
     (d) Upper thoracic catheters can cause Horner's
         syndrome.
     (e) Fluoroscopy can help visualise real-time placement
         of catheter.

19. Epidural stimulation test:
     (a) Low current electrical stimulation is used for
         monitoring and placing catheter.
     (b) Spinal cord stimulation is done for the placement.
     (c) Correct placement is seen with motor stimulation
         with current between 1 and 10 mA.
     (d) Anode is connected to the catheter.
     (e) Current nerve stimulators are ideal for epidural
         stimulation.

20. Paediatric epidural stimulation catheter:
     (a) Metal stylet is required for insertion.
     (b) Muscle twitches should be elicited as catheter is
         advanced.
     (c) The current is transmitted through a conducting fluid.
     (d) Air in the catheter can decrease the stimulation.
     (e) Long catheters may increase the resistance to
         current flow.

21. Epidural ECG technique:
    (a) Can be used with neuromuscular blockade.
    (b) Local anaesthetics in the epidural space augment epidural stimulation.
    (c) The signal from catheter tip is compared with the signal from skin surface.
    (d) T wave changes are seen as the catheter approaches the thoracic region.
    (e) Intrathecal placement is indicated by the loss of the trace.

22. Caudal analgesia:
    (a) A single-shot technique has limited dermatomal spread.
    (b) Size of needle plays an important part in success of blockade.
    (c) Short bevel 22-G needles are better for the blockade.
    (d) Can cause epidermal cell graft tumour in epidural space.
    (e) The needle must be removed before injection.

23. Advantages of caudal anaesthesia:
    (a) Better distribution of local anaesthetic.
    (b) Easier to insert catheter.
    (c) Catheter can be positioned to a higher space.
    (d) Rapid recovery.
    (e) Good post-operative pain management.

24. Caudal epidural block:
    (a) Mostly done in lateral decubitus position.
    (b) Needle insertion is about 70° to parallel.
    (c) Subcutaneous bulging can happen even if the needle is in dural space.
    (d) Swoosh test involves injection of 2.5 ml of saline.
    (e) With catheters, anal motor activity is seen on stimulation with 1–10 mA of current.

25. Caudal epidural block:
    (a) Ultrasound can increase the success.
    (b) Relaxation of anal sphincter signifies successful blockade.
    (c) Ketamine and clonidine can increase the analgesia.
    (d) Epinephrine is contraindicated.
    (e) Skin temperature changes are seen with caudal blockade.

26. Continuous caudal epidural:
    (a) More risk of dural puncture is seen.
    (b) Extension of patient's spine helps in the passage of the catheter.
    (c) Easier insertion is seen in children less than 1 year old.
    (d) Reduced risk of intraosseous injection.
    (e) Injection of normal saline can help in insertion of catheter.

27. Lumbar epidural anaesthesia:
    (a) Usually done after general anaesthesia.
    (b) Loss of resistance to air is preferred in children.
    (c) Distinctive pop may be more easily felt in children.
    (d) Epidural space is shallow in neonates.
    (e) Greater resistance is seen to catheter advancement than adults.

28. Epidural anaesthesia:
    (a) Sympathetic block is well tolerated in children.
    (b) Bolus doses are not normally given in children.
    (c) A mix of opioid and local anaesthetic is not used in children.
    (d) Epidural may cause post-operative delirium in preschool adults.
    (e) Patient-controlled analgesia causes less motor block.

29. Thoracic epidural analgesia:
    (a) Children need higher volume dose of local anaesthetic as compared to adults.
    (b) Paramedian approach is more useful in children.
    (c) Insertion of needle is easier in lower thoracic as compared to higher thoracic level.
    (d) Usually 14- or 16-G needles are used.
    (e) Paramedian approach is more difficult to perform.

30. Spinal anaesthesia in paediatrics:
    (a) Is contraindicated in premature infants.
    (b) Tuffier's line corresponds to L3–L4 interspace.
    (c) Dural sac terminates more caudal in children.
    (d) Cerebrospinal fluid volume is larger in children as compared to adults.
    (e) Sedation used along with spinal anaesthesia may cause bradycardia.

31. Spinal anaesthesia in children:
    (a) Sitting position is preferred.
    (b) Barbotage method is used to decrease false placements of spinal.
    (c) Hypobaric solutions are not used in children.
    (d) Trendelenberg position should be avoided.
    (e) Bromage scale is effective in assessing the block.

32. Complications of spinal anaesthesia:
    (a) Fluid loading prevents hypotension.
    (b) Post-dural puncture headache is seen less in children as compared to the adults.
    (c) Transient neurologic symptoms are not seen.
    (d) Caffeine can be used to treat clonidine induced apnoea.
    (e) An increased intracranial pressure is a contraindication for the spinal block.

33. Indications for spinal anaesthesia:
    (a) Bilateral inguinal hernia repairs in former premature infants.
    (b) Cardiac surgery.
    (c) Post-operative pain relief.
    (d) Increased risk of general anaesthesia.
    (e) Major abdominal surgery.

34. Complications of neuraxial block:
    (a) Pruritus is limited to dermatomes affected by epidural.
    (b) Nausea and vomiting is seen due to stimulation of area postrema.
    (c) Urinary retention seen usually lasts for minutes.
    (d) Respiratory depression has an early and delayed onset.
    (e) Low-dose naloxone does not affect analgesia.

35. Peripheral nerve blocks in children:
    (a) Can be used for chronic pain conditions.
    (b) Ultrasound does not contribute to success in children.
    (c) Less dosage of drugs is required.
    (d) Addition of sodium bicarbonate is painful.
    (e) Doses are different depending upon the additives used.

36. Local anaesthetic doses for blocks:
    (a) Epinephrine is used in concentration of 1:200,000 as an additive.
    (b) Ropivacaine is contraindicated in children.
    (c) Parascalene approach requires more local anaesthetic than adults.
    (d) A volume of 2 ml of local anaesthetic is sufficient for blocks at wrist.
    (e) Children younger than 8 years should not be given bupivacaine 0.5 %.

37. Ilioinguinal nerve block:
    (a) Is the block of choice for hernia surgery.
    (b) Ilioinguinal nerves originates from T12 and L1.
    (c) Nerve pierces internal oblique aponeurosis.
    (d) Perforation of the bowel can occur.
    (e) Femoral nerve block can occur.

38. Rectus sheath block:
    (a) Useful in umbilical surgery.
    (b) Is a block of the tenth intercostal nerve.
    (c) Needle insertion is half cm medial to linea
         semilunaris.
    (d) The solution is deposited anterior to rectus sheath.
    (e) The plane of injection is superficial.

39. Penile nerve block:
    (a) Penis is innervated by pudendal nerve and pelvic
         plexus.
    (b) Epinephrine helps in prolonged blockade.
    (c) Injection is done in subpubic space either side of
         the midline
    (d) Injection is done after penetration of Scarpa's fascia.
    (e) 15 ml of local anaesthetic should be injected for
         effective block.

40. Thoracic paravertebral block:
    (a) Useful for abdominal surgery.
    (b) Mostly done in higher thoracic space.
    (c) Loss of resistance is due to penetration of the
         ligamentum flavum.
    (d) Paravertebral infusions should not be used in the
         paediatric population.
    (e) The block is done in midline.

Answers

1. (a) F   (b) T   (c) T   (d) T   (e) F
   If the child has cognitive ability to understand, consent should be obtained.

2. (a) T   (b) T   (c) F   (d) T   (e) T
   Caudal blockade does not reduce the incidence of post-operative nausea and vomiting. Regional anaesthesia decreases requirement of inhalational agents.

3. (a) T   (b) T   (c) T   (d) T   (e) F
   Myelomeningocele is a relative contraindication.

4. (a) F   (b) T   (c) T   (d) T   (e) T

5. (a) T   (b) F   (c) F   (d) T   (e) T
   Cardiac output is higher in infants than adults (200 ml/kg/min). Most common cause for bradycardia is hypoxia and should be treated with oxygen.

6. (a) T   (b) F   (c) T   (d) F   (e) F
   Brown fat is seen in back, shoulders, legs and around major thoracic vessels. It causes non-shivering thermogenesis. It is deficient in premature infants. Infants loose heat by conduction, convection, evaporation and predominantly by radiation. Neutral thermal environment is one in which oxygen demand, heat loss and energy expenditure are minimal. It is 34 °C for premature babies and 32 and 28 °C for infants and adults, respectively. Platelet function is impaired, but clotting factors are unaffected above 32 °C.

7. (a) T   (b) F   (c) F   (d) T   (e) F

The spinal cord ends at L3 at birth and L12 by 1 year of age. Meninges terminate at the level of S3 at birth and S45 at 1 year. Infants have spongy lobules as opposed to fibrous strands seen in adults. In infants, nerve fibre diameter is smaller with thinner myelin sheaths and increased distance between two nodes, requiring less volume of local anaesthetics. Resistance to epidural blockade of L5–S1 is seen in adults.

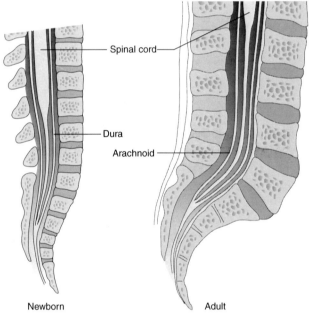

Anatomical differences between infants and adults

8. (a) T   (b) T   (c) T   (d) T   (e) T

Amide local anaesthetics show diminished clearance in neonates and infants younger than 3 months of age until they reach 8 months of age.

9. (a) F   (b) F   (c) F   (d) F   (e) T

Dose is calculated in children on a mg/kg basis. Local anaesthetics are generally associated with negative ionotropic effect on cardiac muscle. It also alters calcium influx leading to decreased myocardial contractility.

10. (a) T   (b) F   (c) T   (d) T   (e) F

Older children can tolerate a higher dose of local anaesthetic as compared to neonates and infants. Bupivacaine is well bound to $\alpha 1$ glycoprotein, and because the levels are lower in neonates, free fraction may increase and cause toxicity. Neurotoxicity is masked by general anaesthetic and cardiotoxicity is seen more.

11. (a) T   (b) F   (c) T   (d) T   (e) T

L enantiomer is seen with fewer side effects.

12. (a) F   (b) T   (c) T   (d) T   (e) T

Effective post-operative pain relief have numerous benefits including earlier ambulation, rapid weaning from ventilators, decreased catabolic state and lower circulating stress hormone levels. Conus medullaris is located at L3 as compared to L1. At 1 year of age, conus medullaris reaches similar level as adults. Caudal catheters are easier to insert because of less densely packed epidural fat.

13. (a) T   (b) F   (c) T   (d) T   (e) T

Body weight is a better correlate than age for predicting spread.

14. (a) T   (b) T   (c) T   (d) T   (e) T

Clonidine is an $\alpha 1$ agonist which acts by stimulating descending noradrenergic medullispinal pathways decreasing the release of nociceptive neurotransmitters in dorsal horn of spinal cord. Epidural midazolam produces analgesia by its effect on GABA receptors in the spinal cord.

15. (a) T   (b) T   (c) F   (d) F   (e) T

Sacral osteomyelitis can be seen with single-shot caudal blocks. Perforation of rectum occurs because of steep angle of needle. Epidural blood patch is effective through formation of gelatinous cover over the dural hole. The dose for blood patch is 0.3 ml/kg body weight.

16. (a) F   (b) T   (c) T   (d) T   (e) T

If the heart rate does not increase with epinephrine-containing solutions, an increase in the blood pressure should raise suspicion of intravascular placement.

17. (a) T   (b) F   (c) T   (d) T   (e) T

The various complications seen are pruritus (26 %), nausea and vomiting (16.9 %) and urinary retention (20.8 %). Incidence of sedation is seen in less than 2 % of patients.

18. (a) F   (b) T   (c) T   (d) T   (e) T

Specificity of ECG changes (>25 % increase in T wave) after the injection of an epinephrine test dose (0.5 μ/kg).

19. (a) T   (b) F   (c) T   (d) F   (e) F

The epidural stimulation test can be used to confirm the epidural placement through stimulation of the spinal nerve roots (not spinal cord) with low electrical stimulation. Cathode lead is connected to epidural catheter, while anode lead is connected to patient's skin. A motor response observed with low-threshold current (<1 mA) suggests intrathecal catheter placement. Most nerve stimulators do not deliver currents >5 mA and are not suitable for epidural stimulation.

20. (a) T   (b) T   (c) T   (d) T   (e) T

    A thin metal stylet is required for effective threading of epidural catheter from a lower spinal level to target upper spinal level. The absence of muscular twitches or resistance to the advancement of catheter may indicate curled or kinked catheter. An ionic solution such as normal saline is used as priming solution.

21. (a) F   (b) F   (c) T   (d) F   (e) F

    The technique cannot be reliably performed if any significant clinical neuromuscular blockade is present. Amplitude of QRS increase as resulting electrode comes closer to thoracic region. The amplitude of QRS is smaller if catheter is in lumbar or sacral region. Intrathecal catheter placement cannot be picked by epidural ECG technique.

22. (a) T   (b) F   (c) T   (d) T   (e) T

    The size of needle or type of needle does not affect the success rate of caudal epidural. Short bevel 22-G needles with stylets offer better tactile sensation when sacrococcygeal ligament is punctured. Styletted needle reduces the risk of epidermal cell graft tumour.

23. (a) T   (b) T   (c) T   (d) T   (e) T

24. (a) T   (b) T   (c) F   (d) F   (e) T

    The block is usually done in lateral position but can be done in prone position. The needle is inserted with an initial angle of 70°, and then the angle is decreased to 20–30° after the sacrococcygeal ligament is pierced. The absence of subcutaneous bulging and lack of resistance upon injection are signs of needle placement. Whoosh test is seen with injection of air with a stethoscope placed over the spine. Swoosh test uses saline.

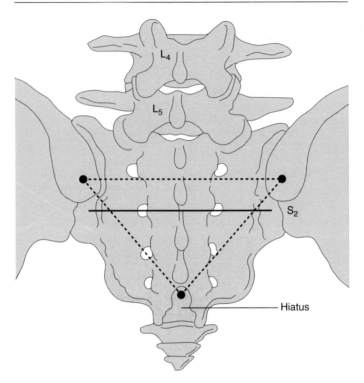

Fig: Landmarks for caudal block

25. (a) T   (b) T   (c) T   (d) F   (e) T

26. (a) T   (b) T   (c) T   (d) T   (e) T

27. (a) T   (b) F   (c) F   (d) T   (e) T
     Air should be avoided due to venous air embolism. The
     ligamentum flavum is less tense so a distinctive pop may
     not be felt.

28. (a) T   (b) F   (c) F   (d) F   (e) T
     A bolus of 0.5–1.0 ml/kg of 0.25 % bupivacaine is given
     to establish block. Most commonly used agents are
     bupivacaine and fentanyl.

29. (a) T (b) F (c) T (d) F (e) T

    Midline approach is more useful in children. 20-G needle is mostly used.

30. (a) F (b) T (c) T (d) T (e) T

    Use of spinal anaesthesia is commonly used in premature infants. Spinal anaesthesia is administered at Tuffier's line in adults which corresponds to L3–L4. Pelvis is small in neonates and infants, and sacrum is located more cephalad, and Tuffier's line crosses vertebral column at L4–L5. Cerebrospinal fluid volume is larger on a ml/kg basis in infants and neonates (4 ml/kg) compared with adults (2 ml/kg).

31. (a) F (b) F (c) T (d) T (e) T

    Spinal anaesthesia is mostly preferred in lateral position. Flexion of head in sitting position may result in airway obstruction. Barbotage method is not used as it may cause high levels of motor blockade and total spinal block. Trendelenberg position should be avoided to avoid total spinal anaesthesia. In children more than 2 years, Bromage scale can be used.

Complete	Unable to move feet or knees
Almost complete	Able to move feet only
Partial	Just able to move knees
None	Full flexion of knees and feet

32. (a) F (b) T (c) F (d) T (e) T

    Fluid preloading does not help in preventing hypotension. Caffeine (10 mg/kg) can be used to treat apnoea caused by clonidine.

33. (a) T (b) T (c) T (d) T (e) T

    Apnoea can occur in former preterm patients following a general anaesthetic, so regional anaesthesia is preferred. Spinal anaesthesia can be used for early extubation in cardiac surgery. Increased risk of general anaesthesia may be seen in syndromes involving laryngomalacia, macroglossia, micrognathia, congenital heart disease and failure to thrive.

34. (a) F (b) T (c) F (d) T (e) T

Pruritus is seen in 20 % of patients after epidural blockade. It is not limited to dermatomal segments affected. Area postrema of 4th ventricle has chemoreceptor trigger zone which causes nausea and vomiting. Urinary retention can persist for 10–20 h and is seen more in males. Early onset of respiratory depression is seen in 1 h after the block and is due to vascular absorption via epidural veins, whereas late phase occurs 6–12 h after the block. Low-dose naloxone (5 μg/kg) reverses complications without reversing analgesia.

35. (a) T (b) F (c) T (d) F (e) T

Peripheral nerve blocks can be used for children with chronic painful conditions like chronic headache, CRPS-1. The dosage required is less because of decrease in α1 acid glycoprotein, allowing free fraction of local anaesthetic. Sodium bicarbonate decreases pain on injection and increases the onset of action of local anaesthetics.

36. (a) T (b) F (c) F (d) T (e) T

Ropivacaine is used both for single-shot injection and continuous infusion.

37. (a) F (b) T (c) T (d) T (e) T

Caudal block is preferred for hernia surgery, but ilioinguinal nerve blocks can be used in relative contraindications to caudal block.

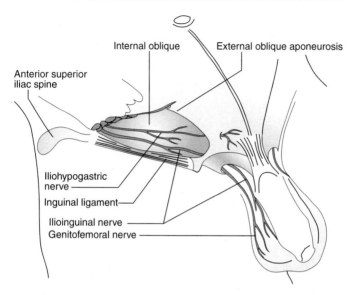

38. (a) T   (b) T   (c) T   (d) F   (e) T

The block is useful in umbilical surgery. The block is of tenth thoracoabdominal intercostals nerve bilaterally. Needle is inserted below umbilicus half centimetres medial to the linea semilunaris. The injection is done between muscle and posterior rectus sheath. The usual depth of injection is 0.5–1.5 cm.

39. (a) T   (b) F   (c) T   (d) T   (e) F

Dorsal nerve of penis supplies shaft of the penis. Epinephrine-containing solutions should not be used for penile block. A maximum of 5 ml should be used.

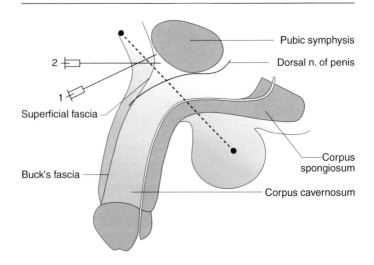

40. (a) T (b) F (c) F (d) F (e) F

    The block is useful for thoracotomies and abdominal
    surgeries. The block is done mostly at T7–T9 level. Loss
    of resistance is seen due to penetration of costo-
    transverse ligament. The needle is inserted 1–2 cm
    lateral to midline. Approximate distance to the space is
    calculated by the formula:

    $20 + (0.5 \times \text{weight in kg})$.

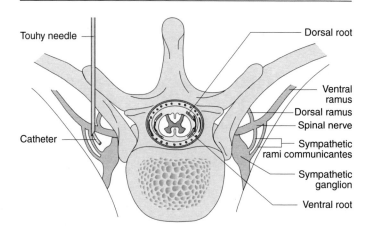

Touhy needle

Dorsal root

Ventral ramus

Dorsal ramus

Spinal nerve

Sympathetic rami communicantes

Catheter

Sympathetic ganglion

Ventral root

Further Reading

Allman KG, Wilson IH (2006) Oxford handbook of anaesthesia, 2nd edn. Oxford University Press

Chelly JE (2004) Peripheral nerve block: a color atlas, 2nd edn. Lippincott Williams and Wilkins

Hadzic A (2007) Textbook of regional anesthesia and acute pain management. New York school of regional anaesthesia. McGraw-Hill Medical

Jankovic D (2004) Regional nerve blocks and infiltration therapy, 3rd edn. Blackwell Publishing Ltd

Neal JM, Rathmell JP (2007) Complications in regional anaesthesia and pain medicine. Saunders, Elsevier

Prithvi Raj P (2003) Textbook of regional anaesthesia. Churchill Livingstone

R. Gupta, D. Patel, *Multiple Choice Questions in Regional Anaesthesia*,
DOI 10.1007/978-3-642-31257-1, © Springer-Verlag Berlin Heidelberg 2013